BRIGHT LINE Eating

Hay House Titles of Related Interest

YOU CAN HEAL YOUR LIFE, the movie, starring Louise Hay & Friends
(available as a 1-DVD program, an expanded 2-DVD set,
and an online streaming video)
Learn more at www.hayhouse.com/louise-movie

THE SHIFT, the movie, starring Dr. Wayne W. Dyer
(available as a 1-DVD program, an expanded 2-DVD set,
and an online streaming video)
Learn more at www.hayhouse.com/the-shift-movie

ⓞⓞⓞ

INTEGRATIVE WELLNESS RULES: A Simple Guide to Healthy Living,
by Dr. Jim Nicolai

*MIRACLES NOW: 108 Life-Changing Tools for Less Stress, More Flow,
and Finding Your True Purpose,* by Gabrielle Bernstein

RECOVERY 2.0: Move Beyond Addiction and Upgrade Your Life,
by Tommy Rosen

*SECRETS OF MEDITATION: A Practical Guide to Inner Peace
and Personal Transformation,* by davidji

All of the above are available at your local bookstore,
or may be ordered by visiting:

Hay House USA: www.hayhouse.com®
Hay House Australia: www.hayhouse.com.au
Hay House UK: www.hayhouse.co.uk
Hay House India: www.hayhouse.co.in

BRIGHT LINE Eating

The Science of Living Happy, Thin, and Free

Susan Peirce Thompson, Ph.D.

HAY HOUSE, INC.
Carlsbad, California • New York City
London • Sydney • New Delhi

Published in the United States by: Hay House, Inc.: www.hayhouse.com® • *Published in Australia by: Hay House Australia Pty. Ltd.:* www.hayhouse.com. au • *Published in the United Kingdom by:* Hay House UK, Ltd.: www.hayhouse. co.uk • *Published in India by: Hay House Publishers India:* www.hayhouse.co.in

Cover design: Amy Grigoriou
Interior design: Nick C. Welch
Interior illustrations: Cinzia Damonte
Indexer: Laura Ogar

Library of Congress Cataloging-in-Publication Data

Thompson, Susan Peirce, author.
Title: Bright line eating : the science of living happy, thin, and free / Susan Peirce Thompson, Ph.D.
Description: 1st edition. | Carlsbad, California : Hay House, Inc., 2017. | Includes bibliographical references.
Identifiers: LCCN 2016040447 | ISBN 9781401952532 (hardback)
Subjects: LCSH: Weight loss--Popular works. | Exercise--Popular works. | Self-care, Health--Popular works. | BISAC: HEALTH & FITNESS / Weight Loss. | HEALTH & FITNESS / Diets. | HEALTH & FITNESS / Exercise.
Classification: LCC RM222.2 .T4853 2017 | DDC 613.2/5--dc23 LC record available at https://lccn.loc.gov/2016040447

Hardcover ISBN: 978-1-4019-5253-2

14 13 12 11 10 9 8 7
1st edition, March 2017

Printed in the United States of America

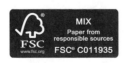

For David

And for you

CONTENTS

PART V:
Goal Weight, Maintenance, and Beyond

FOREWORD

BY JOHN ROBBINS

I've been advocating for healthy food choices for more than three decades. As a best-selling author and the President of the Food Revolution Network, I've had the great privilege of helping millions of people to improve their diets and, in many cases, turn their health and their lives around.

Over these years, I've seen many people become inspired to eat in a new way. Some of them succeeded and experienced health outcomes beyond their wildest dreams. But many others struggled to sustain food choices that they knew were in their own best interests. Despite having plenty of knowledge and will-power, they found themselves succumbing to addictive pulls. Despite their best intentions, they watched their health, and even their self-esteem, degrade in the process.

A question began to burn inside me. Why is it that, when it comes to food, so many people are unable to consistently act in their own best interests? Why is it that so many accomplished, caring, and intelligent people are eating their way to misery and premature death?

As a neuroscientist, Susan Peirce Thompson has spent decades studying this problem. Stunningly, incredibly, I believe she has actually cracked the code.

Susan also walks (and eats) her talk. She is among the less than one-tenth of 1 percent of the population that has gone from being obese to slender and kept that weight off for more than ten years.

She's an Adjunct Associate Professor of Brain and Cognitive Sciences at the University of Rochester, President of the Institute for Sustainable Weight Loss, and founder and CEO of Bright Line Eating Solutions. She's dedicated her life to helping people achieve the vibrant health and zest for life that can accompany permanent weight loss. The operative word being permanent. Because, shockingly, there is not a single peer-reviewed scientific journal article that shows ANY weight loss program taking ANY cohort of overweight people and helping them to get down to a healthy weight and *stay there*.

But if you look at Bright Line Eating's data, you see that Susan has had a level of success that is nothing short of spectacular.

In 2015 and 2016 my 350,000-member-strong network collaborated with Susan in putting on a pair of eight-week courses. Between the two courses we had 5,600 participants, the vast majority of whom joined the program hoping to lose weight. In eight weeks, they combined to lose more than 90,000 pounds.

When I see these kinds of results, 90,000 pounds lost in eight weeks, I'm floored. And all the more so because I know that those numbers, as impressive as they are, do not include the substantial amount of additional weight participants continued to lose after the eight-week programs ended.

And these are not just numbers to me. I think, with gratitude, of the many cases of diabetes that have been averted. I think, with thankfulness, of the many heart attacks and cases of cancer that have been prevented. I think, with joy, of all the people who are now more present in their lives, because they feel more confident in their bodies, and who can show up more fully for the people they love.

Of course, most weight-loss programs promise the moon. But the only one I'm aware of that even begins to achieve this level of success is Susan's. In fact, the contrast with other weight-loss programs is not just striking. It's staggering.

Here's what the preliminary data show: it appears that people in Susan's programs lose two-and-a-half times more weight, and they do so seven times faster than people in the country's most popular weight-loss program.

And unlike that program, the Bright Line Eating business model is not based on recidivism. It's based on people reaching their goal weight and sustaining that weight—living "Happy, Thin, and Free."

Recently, I led a retreat at a hot springs healing resort in Oregon. Among the attendees were eight people who had taken Susan's course. I invited them to tell the group how much weight, if any, they had lost using her program. I did not know if they would choose to answer. Nor did I have any idea, if they did, what they would say.

All of them chose to answer. And this is exactly what they said:

"Forty-five pounds."

"Sixty pounds."

"Seventy-five pounds."

"Thirty-five pounds."

"Fifty pounds."

"Eighty pounds."

"Sixty-five pounds."

"Forty pounds."

As these people spoke, they were smiling from ear to ear. Every one of them looked radiant, vibrant, and happy.

In the last few years, I've had the great pleasure of getting to know Susan Peirce Thompson as a colleague, and as a friend. Now, through this book, you will have the great good fortune of getting to know her and her amazing work.

Congratulations. You are about to meet one of the most brilliant and extraordinary people on this earth. And if you are someone who has struggled with weight issues, you may very well be about to meet the answer to your prayers.

THE OBESITY EPIDEMIC: NOT A PROBLEM, A MYSTERY IN PLAIN SIGHT

Something is awry.

Over the past half century or so, there's been a shift in how our bodies and brains react to food. As a consequence, as a species we are getting fatter, and no amount of education or effort seems to be helping.

The statistics are as bad as you think. Roughly *2 billion* people worldwide are now overweight, and 600 million of them are obese.[1] In the United States alone, 108 million people are on a diet. That number comes from *The U.S. Weight Loss and Diet Control Market,*[2] which merely measures people actively spending money on diet-related products and services. It doesn't count all the people trying to eat less or get healthier on their own.

And it's not just an American issue. Obesity is now a bigger problem in developing nations than malnutrition.[3] The Middle East has some of the highest per capita rates of Type 2 diabetes in the world: 20 percent of the adult population.[4] The combination of a hot climate, prohibition on alcohol, and high disposable income results in people drinking bottled soft drinks—sometimes four or five sodas a day. *Boom.* Type 2 diabetes.[5]

The consequences of this problem couldn't be more dire: 63 percent of people die prematurely from diet-related diseases including heart disease, cancer, diabetes, and stroke.[6] Over the next 20 years, the World Economic Forum estimates that developed nations will spend *$47 trillion* on diseases caused by the global-industrial diet.[7] We are eating ourselves sick—and into the poorhouse.

But here's the statistic that I want to focus on: among the obese who try to lose weight, the failure rate is 99 percent. Literally. Ninety-nine percent do not succeed at getting slim.[8] And for that precious 1 percent who do succeed, the triumph is temporary. The vast majority regain the weight over the next few years. The average dieter spends a whole lot of money and makes *four or five new attempts* each year,[9] with almost no hope of success.

This is all truly bizarre. Maybe we're not seeing it because we've become inured to the hopelessness of the struggle. Let's consider if this happened in a different domain: If colleges and universities only graduated 1 percent of their students, and researchers found that the other 99 percent of students were dropping out and reenrolling four and five times each year while spending billions of dollars to do it, that would be front-page news. We would be outraged. We would say something smelled fishy, and we'd demand that it be fixed. We certainly wouldn't be thinking that the 99 percent were probably just lazy or weak-willed.

No, there's something strange going on here, and we're clearly missing important pieces of the puzzle. I think that we can all agree—and the research is very clear—that people are genuinely motivated to lose weight.[10] They're spending enormous sums of money to do it. Few things are more desirable in our Western culture than being slender. So why can't people succeed?

When I was overweight, I wanted to get thin with every fiber of my being. I was desperate to get that weight off. I remember the focus and intention I would put into each new attempt—I was always so sure that I would finally make it work. I would weigh myself, measure myself, write down my goals, stay up late reading about the food plan I was going to start, and then commence with fanfare and tons of enthusiasm. And it *would* work! I'd start to lose weight! Then . . . there would be some kind of *Twilight Zone* time warp and, a few months later, I would be even fatter than before and rallying the effort for yet another attempt.

What happened between point A and point B? And why was I not really online and aware of the unraveling of that attempt?

Let's go back to that fact about the 99 percent of people who fail to lose all their excess weight. First, it's strange that people are failing so badly. Second, *it's strange that we're not noticing that it's strange.* It's bizarre that this phenomenon is happening right under our noses and nobody is noticing. Why doesn't anybody seem to wonder why smart, capable, educated, successful, motivated people who really want to get slender just can't do it?

I really want us, as a society, to understand that we do not have an obesity *problem.* We have an obesity *mystery.* The problem itself doesn't make any sense. There's no other field of endeavor that I'm aware of where intelligence, determination, talent, and capability have so little bearing on the outcome.

When I was trying to lose weight, it totally baffled me that I couldn't do it—because I was capable in so many other areas. I had earned a Ph.D. in Brain and Cognitive Sciences. I had good friends, and I was happily married. I ran a marathon. I was fat when I ran that marathon, but I ran it nonetheless. I couldn't even jog to the mailbox when I first started, but I put my mind to it and, with some friends in graduate school, we trained hard and did it. We ran a 26.2-mile marathon without taking a single walking step. And I lost 10 pounds. I had 60 pounds to lose, but I merely lost 10 of them. Exercise is not the answer.

What is?

That's what I'm going to explain in this book. I'm going to present you with information on how the brain blocks weight loss, and what exactly you can do about it.

There *is* a solution. Thousands of people in my Bright Line Eating Boot Camps have used this method to lose weight—collectively over 300,000 pounds so far—and the number who have lost *all* their excess weight and are *keeping it off* continues to rise. I am talking about people who have lived their entire adult lives excessively overweight who are now thin—something they never imagined was ever going to be possible for them.

Bright Line Eating gave them hope again. It delivered on the promise.

It solved the mystery.

I wrote this book because I want everyone to have that solution. The information contained in these pages is vital to changing our cultural understanding of what being overweight is—*not* a willpower deficit and *not* a moral shortcoming—rather, the by-product of a brain hijacked by modern food. And, more crucially, I want to show you what a solution that works actually looks like. It's not about six small meals a day, free days, or even lots of exercise. I will teach you about Bright Lines, automaticity, and support. Bright Lines are clear, unambiguous boundaries that you just don't cross, like a nonsmoker just doesn't smoke. They work because they align with how the brain works.

No one should have to suffer in a body that doesn't bring them joy. No one should spend a single additional minute feeling like a failure because conventional diets that don't work with our brain chemistry fail them.

If you've almost given up attempting to lose weight because you're exhausted from trying so hard and not succeeding, if your health has become an issue and you've got to make a change, or if you just have a few pounds to lose and really would like to shed them and *keep them off*, then I have good news. You can learn why your brain has been blocking you from losing weight and adopt a simple system that will permanently turn that around.

You no longer have to feel lost in a flood of confusing and contradictory information on how to eat. Or languish on the couch, overeating late into the evening, knowing you're choosing suicide on the installment plan. Or feel like your weight is holding you back from finally living your dreams and being the person you were meant to be.

Get ready to take back control of your brain and live your life as you never have before—*Happy, Thin, and Free.*

MY STORY

Let me tell you a story. While sometimes colorful around the edges, I actually think it represents, at its core, the garden-variety suffering of millions of people who are overweight, hooked on food, and desperate for a solution.

After all I've lived through, I can say this: I have a very addictable brain. At one time or another I've been on the merry-go-round with just about every addictive substance on the planet, and nothing, I mean *nothing* is harder to kick than food.

The Beginning

One of my earliest memories from childhood is being given two marshmallows. I might have been four. My parents, two avowed hippies, were recently divorced and scraping together a living in San Francisco—he as a taxi driver, she in a small shop at Fisherman's Wharf selling imported alpaca sweaters and rugs they'd discovered on their motorcycle travels through South America. They both worked long hours trying to provide for me, and this was especially true during summers, when the shop stayed open until 9 P.M. During those long, hot months I was often flown to stay with family friends on Sunshine Mesa in Colorado. I loved the horses, the ponds, and the fort on the side of the hill; I loved the attention I received from my parents' friends, who hadn't been able to have children of their own yet. But mostly I loved those marshmallows. I can remember the feel of them in my little hands, the powdery smell, the sunlight setting them aglow in my eagerly outstretched palms.

Before long, I realized that they lived in the cabinet. That when the adults were out feeding the animals, I could drag a chair over to the counter, climb up, and surreptitiously help myself. This is my first memory of feeling compelled to eat more than I knew the adults around me would condone, and the beginning of a long journey of hiding, sneaking, and stealing food. What they offered outright I also took full advantage of: on errand day I'd jump to volunteer, slogging through a day of buying feed and standing around in the relentless heat because I knew at some point we'd visit a store that sold candy. One day in town, I got a finger waggled in my face and a grown-up said, "You be careful, young missy. You're a sugar addict." I didn't really know exactly what that was, but somehow I knew it fit.

Once I got a little older, I became a latchkey kid. A latchkey kid who knew how to cook. By the age of eight, I could have made you Thanksgiving dinner, single-handedly, with all the dishes arriving hot to the table at the right time. On my mom's side of the family there were true gourmets: my grandma Polly was a friend of Julia Child's and she and my uncle Hafe would discuss the *Larousse Gastronomique* over wine at a dinner party and debate whether it was acceptable to use a white onion in place of a shallot in an emergency. I was proud that I didn't eat out of bags or boxes, that I cooked *from scratch*. But what started as a love of baking and sharing time in the kitchen with my mom turned, by age nine, into an obsession with raw cookie dough. I would come home from school and make a full batch with no pretense of baking it. I'd just sit on the floor in front of the TV with the bowl in my lap, eat until I felt sick, and then rush to clean it all up before my mother got home.

My mom was less into fancy food than healthy food. She loved astrology, yoga, and throwing the I Ching, and through her influence I grew up on the nutritional philosophies of Adelle Davis and Nathan Pritikin. The first time we decided together to really *do* the Pritikin Diet, I was maybe ten. Neither of us had weight to lose at that point—it was just about being maximally healthy. I remember feeling empowered and excited, but I don't remember it lasting long.

Right around that time, I experienced my first episode of serious depression. I was back at Sunshine Mesa, but, unlike previous summers, I wasn't enjoying myself. I didn't want to pick cherries, trap grasshoppers in a jar, or do any of the things I usually loved. All I wanted to do was sleep. Everyone thought I was homesick, but long, tortured calls to my mom didn't help. We all breathed a sigh of relief when summer was over and I got to fly back home to San Francisco.

When I was twelve years old, I decided to go off sugar. I remember being excited about it and thinking carefully about what I would count as "sugar." Would I eat honey? Maple syrup? Yogurt with fruit on the bottom? I drew a strict line and declared that if something even *tasted* sweet I wouldn't eat it. Looking back, I now see that as my first Bright Line. It stayed bright for longer than two months, and the main thing I remember about that time was that I felt *great*. Totally empowered. And then one day I was pulled in by a scintillating, sugary treat . . . I debated, telling myself that surely I'd been virtuous for long enough. I ate it. Thus ended the no-sugar experiment.

A year later, a new factor was thrown into the mix: puberty. And with it came body dissatisfaction. Somehow I'd made it to the age of thirteen without really being concerned about my weight or my shape, but after puberty that all changed. I was only fifteen pounds overweight, but I carried it all around my middle and, compared to my petite little mom, I felt enormous. From then on though, any further attempts at dieting were thwarted by my depression and isolation. In school, I was out of sync with my peers because my IQ tested high for someone twice my age, yet my social skills lagged way behind. I felt different and rejected. Food was my companion, my excitement, and, oftentimes, my only friend. But, I think, even had none of those things been true, my brain would still have been hard-wired for addiction. Now. More. Again.

Spiraling Down

My dopamine receptors were primed to need more than I could get from food. In the midst of my adolescent explorations, I found the only diet that ever seemed to really work: drugs. When I was fourteen, a friend from summer camp offered me mushrooms at a UB40 concert. Against my better judgment, I tried them. We explored Tilden Park and then drove around until the sun came up. I had never felt so free, so connected with the universe, so effortlessly at home with other people. I collapsed into bed and when I awoke, 20 hours later, I padded across the hall to the bathroom and stepped on the scale. *I had lost seven pounds.* My world tilted on its axis.

I was hooked.

Over the next six years, my life slowly spiraled out of control. My stellar grade-school education came in handy: I was able to maintain a 4.0 with minimal effort and scanty attendance. Whenever my parents confronted me about my late nights or money that had gone missing from my grandmother's purse, I just countered by telling them my grades were great, my life was on track, I was *fine*.

I was so *not* fine.

Anything new I was introduced to, I wanted more of: acid, ecstasy, cigarettes, alcohol, sex. There was never such a thing as "enough." And when the drug dealer wouldn't answer his pager, when there was no money for nicotine, no fake ID to buy alcohol, there was always a big bowl of pasta or cookie dough to take the edge off. My weight continued to plague me.

Then, in the fall of my senior year, when I should have been in AP Chemistry class, I met a guy playing pool in the middle of the day. We became inseparable and within the first week he offered me my first hit of crystal meth.

That was it. I had found my solution.

Suddenly, I could go *days* without getting hungry. Beyond not being hungry, I had *zero* interest in food. And I finally got thin.

It was magical.

Of course, I may have been *thin*, but I most definitely was not *well*. My guidance counselor saw me spinning away from my future, away from hope, and pulled me out of class one day and insisted that I fill out some paperwork for a program at UC Berkeley, a prestigious school, but also my local state school. Because of my accelerated test scores, I would automatically be admitted as a freshman in the fall if I could just graduate from high school and pass one class on the Berkeley campus during my senior year. At the time, when he shoved the papers under my nose, I scoffed at how little I thought I'd need them—I still assumed Harvard was in my future and had no idea how far drugs were about to take me from my path. Looking back, all I can say is, "Thank God."

Things were crumbling fast. I couldn't seem to get out of bed to go to class anymore. But dropping out would nix my acceptance to Berkeley. So I found a loophole: I could take an equivalency test. Which I did—on acid—and passed. And somehow I managed to get myself across the bridge to Berkeley and pass that one mandatory class as well: Introduction to Sociology. So I left a wedge in the door to my future, then ran in the other direction.

I decided that all my problems were America's fault and I moved to Canada. To which I can only say to my eighteen-year-old self: *o-kay.* On the plus side, disconnected from my "community" back home, I did manage to get myself off crystal meth. Hold your applause. I was in no way sober yet, and over the cold, dark months I stayed inside and gained forty pounds. By smoking cigarettes and eating . . . wait for it . . . granola. I smoked cartons and cartons of cigarettes and ate boxes and boxes of granola. Finally, I realized my mistake and returned to California. By that point, my mother had sold her struggling shop and moved down to San Jose. I moved in with her and tried to assemble the fragments of my life into something that felt like it had some purpose, some direction.

So I enrolled in San Jose City College and got a job at a movie theater, selling popcorn. The theater's manager would freebase cocaine after work, and I wanted to try it. I knew it was dangerous, but I figured I'd been successful at kicking crystal meth so I could handle myself. Within mere weeks, I graduated to smoking crack. The weight poured off, I felt like myself again, and I left my mom in San Jose and thought I'd have a fun summer back up in San Francisco.

It got worse from there. As I sank deeper and deeper into the abyss of the underworld, I funded my habit exactly the way you imagine a reckless nineteen-year-old girl might. I managed never to have to sleep outside, but, having exhausted everyone's good graces, I was homeless. Everyone around me was using substances, or using me, and I had shut out the people who loved me most.

Shortly after my twentieth birthday, on a Tuesday morning in August, I finally hit bottom. I was in a seedy hotel in a slum on South Van Ness Avenue. I'd been there, smoking crack, for days. In one clear and poignant moment, I had a vision of who I'd become—it contrasted sharply with my childhood dreams of getting an Ivy League education and contributing something important to the world. Suddenly, I knew that if I didn't get up and get out of there *right then*, I would never become anything more than I was at that moment. I got my jacket and walked out the door.

I went to a friend's apartment; he graciously let me in to sleep and shower. Refreshed, I put my pager on my hip, ready to go back to work. But, as fate would have it, I had scheduled a date for that night with a cute guy who'd chatted me up at a gas station at 3 A.M. several days prior. Miraculously, despite the chaos in my life, I kept the date. Miraculously, instead of dinner and a movie, the "first date" he decided to take me on turned out to be a 12-Step meeting for alcohol and drug addiction. Miraculously, I have abstained from drugs and alcohol since that blessed day, August 9, 1994, a date that will forever be ingrained in my brain.

I committed to my recovery as fervently as I'd taken to addiction. I went to meetings daily, completed the year at San Jose

City College, finally reenrolled at UC Berkeley, and graduated two years later summa cum laude with a 4.0 and a major in cognitive science. After my years of addiction, you could not have presented me with a more fascinating topic to study. I wanted to know how the brain worked and why one like mine could go so far off the rails. My in-depth study of the brain's reactions to food would come later, but the core curiosity began there.

Academically, I had my life back on track. I had rebuilt trust with my family. But if you think we're anywhere close to a happy ending, I am guessing you have no idea what it's like to live under the tyranny of food addiction.

Nowhere Near Free

Of the thousands of students at Berkeley, *I* was selected to give the student keynote address at graduation for my division. It was an enormous honor, one that I had clawed my way back from the brink to deserve. My parents were bursting with pride. But instead of being excited on graduation day, I was kneeling beside my bed, crying.

Why?

Because I was fat.

I'd known when I quit drugs that I would gain a ton of weight, but I'd forgotten how torturous it was to have to show up places in a body that just made me want to hide. Losing weight sounded great in theory, but every time I sat down to write a paper, I brought along a bowl of comfort food for support. Sometimes that "comfort food" was simply a box of brown sugar and a spoon.

One evening at dusk, I stood on a hill looking down at the campus and the twinkly Golden Gate Bridge beyond, feeling utterly drained and exhausted, as if I had hundred-pound weights strapped to my ankles, and thought *this is what being poisoned feels like.* And then I reached into the pocket of my oversized coat, pulled out a marshmallow, and ate it. I did it again thirty seconds later, and thirty seconds after that. I couldn't stop. I couldn't even slow. Each time I tried to control my eating, it would culminate in a binge. Yes, my addiction to drugs had taken me to more dangerous places, but my addiction to food was proving to be even more painful—and much more insidious. It hid in plain sight. I couldn't have snorted lines of meth in the middle of campus, but no one called campus security when I ate those marshmallows.

I graduated and managed to make the cross-country move to the University of Rochester, in New York, where leading research in the field of brain and cognitive sciences was being done. As soon as I got there, I fell in love with the work and with the community in my department, but control was gradually slipping beyond my reach. Overcome by the bleak, sunless winters, I started sleeping until late afternoon with laundry and dirty dishes piling up around me. My bingeing escalated, as did my attempts to lose weight. At one time or another I tried them all: Fit for Life, Body-for-LIFE, the Pritikin Diet (again and again), Susan Powter's Stop the Insanity, the USANA Lean program, Weight Watchers (multiple times), the Raquel Welch Total Beauty and Fitness Program, the Atkins Diet, Dexatrim, mindful eating, and Ellyn Satter's Competent Eating. I read Geneen Roth books and tried listening to my body. I lifted weights, ran a marathon, went to personal therapy, group therapy, and hypnosis. I tried forgetting about losing weight and just focusing on loving myself more. And I attended endless, *endless* 12-Step food meetings. Sometimes I'd march my binge foods out to the dumpster and throw them away with finality, pouring vinegar all over them lest I be tempted to come back to retrieve them later. But I could never seem to make the resolve *last*.

One week in November, I binged so hard that an inflammatory fluid built up in my knees and the next morning I couldn't stand up. I called my dad, and he got me on a plane back to California and booked an appointment with a well-respected eating disorder specialist.

She kindly and gently explained that the usual signals the brain sends to tell us to stop eating didn't work for me—that my brain was wired differently. She showed me a pair of graphs from of a recently published research article. One of the graphs showed a straight line. She said, "When a normal eater sits down to eat a meal, she starts off hungry and gradually gets full." And then she pointed to the other graph, which showed a U-shaped curve. She said, "When you sit down to eat a meal, you start off hungry, gradually get fuller, but then, midway through the meal, you start to get hungrier again, so that by the end of the meal you're just as hungry as you were when you started."

That made so much sense to me! I never seemed to get full. At the end of the appointment, she sent me on my way with a prescription for a very high dose of an antidepressant medication that she said would also help my eating compulsion.

It didn't.

So I prescribed my own course of treatment, one that I knew *would* work: bulimia.

A year later I met my husband, David. He was unconditionally accepting and supportive, oftentimes having more faith than I did that I was going to beat this. We got married, bought a little house right near campus, and blended his dog and my three cats into one big family. But soon we noticed that our newlywed habit of eating in restaurants all the time had expanded our waistlines—mine more than his. I didn't know it at the time, but I'd officially crossed an invisible but significant line. I was obese.

We committed to a bikini-body challenge. We looked each other in the eye and swore that we would stay 100 percent committed and complete the 12-week challenge together. The plan included six days a week of prescribed meals and exercise. Sunday was a "free" day, when you could eat whatever you wanted. We followed the program strictly, and within weeks David was back to being the lean-and-fit guy he had been when we met. I, on the other hand, was going crazy. On the free day, while David ate his one burger, an order of fries, and a small dish of ice cream—just something to check that "indulgence" box and get back to the routine Monday morning—I would eat everything that wasn't nailed down. And the rest of the week, the obsession was deafening. *On Wednesday we're having friends over for dinner and I want to cook something amazing, so I think I'll transfer half my free day to Wednesday. But then on Sunday, if I can't stop eating halfway through the day, I'll have blown it. But I can do some extra exercise and get off those calories and I'll be okay—unless I won't have time to both exercise and drive to all the different restaurants and stores I'll need to visit to get all the food I'll want to eat before midnight comes and my free day is over. And if the end of my free day comes and I've forgotten to eat something I really meant to eat, I'll have to wait a whole week so I'd better . . .* and onandonandonandon. I was supposed to be focusing on my dissertation, but I only had one radio station playing in my head, and it was tuned to "all food all the time." Something about toggling between six days of control and what I was doing to my body on Sundays was mentally undoing me. The plan wasn't working for me. I had to give it up.

Not only was I sickeningly disappointed in myself, but I felt I had let David down, too. I had broken my word. It was clear to both of us that I was powerless over my relationship with food.

But I also had my first clue. Something knocked at the researcher in my brain. Why did the "free" day work for David, but undo me? How exactly—quantifiably—were we different?

I didn't have the answer yet, but I was finally asking the right question.

Bright Lines

I had been going to 12-Step meetings for compulsive eaters since the fall of 1995, and while the community support had been profoundly helpful in terms of making me feel less alone, they weren't helping me get better—it was now 2003 and I was just as miserable as ever. For one thing, my food plan was left entirely up to me, so inevitably I stayed hooked on sugar and flour. Desperate from the disappointment of failing—not only the bikini-body challenge, but, it felt like, my marriage—I found another 12-Step food program that did offer specific guidance about what to eat.

I went to my first meeting on a Wednesday night in late May and decided to give it a try. Lo and behold, *it worked*. Within a few short months I had a slender physique, a spring in my step, and joy bursting in my heart. I was finally free!

I was sure I'd found the solution to the world's obesity epidemic, and I worked hard at spreading the word. Over time, though, I started doubting that this was a solution for the masses. First of all, I was being told the program should come before family. Second, my meetings, phone calls, and service obligations—all part of the program—consumed more than 20 hours a week. And finally, there was a maddening arbitrariness and lack of scientific basis to many of the requirements and food rules. For example, at various times, by various sponsors, I was told I couldn't eat soup, nuts, seeds, corn, peas, cherries, mangoes, grapes, beans, lentils, veggie burgers, or even mixed vegetables—they weren't "simple" enough. My husband got tired of it all and suddenly began questioning whether he wanted to stay married to me. Literally. I found a new sponsor and that helped a bit, but he remained concerned on several fronts. My husband wasn't the only one put off by the intensive process. Only a minute fraction of the people I knew who needed to lose weight were willing to even give it a try. I didn't believe it then, but I can see now that this 12-Step program was a good fit for only a very small segment of the population. Nevertheless, I remain eternally grateful to it. It provided exactly what I needed at the time: a mandate not to eat sugar or flour. *Ever.*

Once I was finally, truly "off" sugar and flour, my brain still took months to heal. The damage to my dopamine receptors was extreme, so they didn't just spring back into action. It wasn't spontaneous, but gradually the world did come back into color. Miraculously, the depression that had plagued me on and off since childhood disappeared completely and I got off my antidepressants for good. I was thin. I was sober. I could think. I could function.

I finished my dissertation. We moved to Australia, where I had landed a two-year postdoctoral research and teaching fellowship in psychology at the University of New South Wales. After it ended, we moved back to America and I became a tenured psychology professor. I started teaching a course on the psychology of eating. I returned again to the question I had asked back when I gave up the bikini-body challenge—what was different about how my brain reacted to unstructured eating and how David's brain did? I immersed myself in researching the neuroscience and psychology of truly sustainable weight loss.

I also began working with many people one-on-one, helping them to lose their excess weight and keep it off. Personally, I survived without the crutch of excess food through infertility treatments, extremely premature twins, a second surprise pregnancy, and all the other ups and downs of life on life's terms.

Fast-forward many years to a cold January morning. It was 5 A.M. and, as per my usual morning routine, I was meditating. As I sat silently on my meditation bench there appeared, in my heart and mind, a big, clear mandate: write the book, *Bright Line Eating*. The information I had in my head could help so many; it needed to be shared. It could help change our cultural weight-loss narrative from one of "moderation" and "control" to one of *Bright Lines* and *freedom*. I had been through the wringer; through years and years of pain and over 20 years watching thousands succeed or fail in various kinds of food programs, I knew what *didn't* work and why, I knew what *did* work and why, and I was lucky to have the academic background that allowed me to connect the dots. I could explain the science behind it all. I know there are millions of overweight and unhealthy people suffering in the world, praying for a solution. In the stillness that morning, I throbbed with their prayers and their need. The solution had to get out.

The trouble was, my life was already completely full. After my daily 5 A.M. meditation session, I was then on the phone for 90 minutes, taking back-to-back 15-minute phone calls and food commitments from the myriad people I was helping to lose weight. Then David and I had to get our three little kids ready for daycare and school. And then I went off to work, teaching college courses and mentoring students.

But I felt this book had to be written. So the very next morning, I started rising at 4:25 A.M. to write my book proposal—*before* morning meditation. I was diligent and made progress, but as the weeks unfolded I found out that, in order for the book to have the reach that I hoped it would, I needed to build a "platform" first. I couldn't imagine finding the time to start a podcast or go on speaking tours. The only platform I could envision fitting into my life was an e-mail newsletter. I vowed to write an e-mail once or twice a week that would help people understand the psychology and neuroscience of truly sustainable weight loss. So I did that.

On August 5th, I launched it. By the end of the year, it had 800 subscribers. Six months later it had 10,000. Six months after that, 100,000. And after another six months, 200,000. In short, the list grew from nothing to over 200,000 subscribers in less than two years, which is unusual in the extreme. And as the community grew, their needs grew. I began offering what I called Boot Camps. The first Boot Camp had 40 people. I taught the material on live conference calls in the evenings after tucking my three daughters into bed and grading my college students' papers. Soon the online Boot Camp registrations grew to thousands of people and I created a full online course with video tutorials. It became clear that I could no longer be a professor *and* serve the needs of this burgeoning movement. What was I to do? I had envisioned being a college professor until retirement. But Bright Line Eating was helping so many people, relieving so much misery. The mandate to grow the movement couldn't be ignored. So I handed back tenure and dove all in.

I hired a team, and together we started a research program to track the results we were seeing in the Boot Camps. From the research responses, we know that the average Boot Camper, in 8 weeks, loses 19 pounds. Many lose much more, and keep going all the way to goal weight. As of the final editing of this book, we've helped people from over 75 countries lose over 300,000 pounds. We believe Bright Line Eating is the most successful weight-loss program on earth, and we are amassing data that backs that up.

With this data collection effort and the success of the Bright Line Eating program, a new opportunity emerged. I was invited to become an Adjunct Associate Professor of Brain and Cognitive Sciences at the University of Rochester, my grad school alma mater. We are mapping out an ambitious research agenda, the outline of which is laid out in Chapter Fifteen at the conclusion of this book.

Just recently, my Bright Line Eating team and I set what we call our Everest Goal. It's big and outrageous, but I think we'll do it. By 2040, or before, we want to help *one million people* get all the way down to goal weight and stay there, permanently. One million people finally living Happy, Thin, and Free.

It's been a wild ride, but at its core it's pretty simple. The modern diet wires our brain to work *against* us, but we can rewire it to work *for* us. We are not weak. We are not stupid. We are simply trapped on a chemical hamster wheel and haven't been given the tools to get off. Until now.

In Part I of this book, I will give you all the science you need to understand what is happening inside your brain that is blocking your weight loss, and how the Standard American Diet hijacks our hormones and neurotransmitters, leaving us with insatiable hunger, overpowering cravings, and vulnerable to something I call the Willpower Gap.

Then, in Part II, I will explain how Bright Line Eating solves those problems by literally rewiring your brain to work *with* your goals, not against them. I will introduce you to the Four Bright Lines that will change your life and end your dieting cycle forever: Sugar, Flour, Meals, and Quantities. And I'll give you the formula for integrating them into your life in a way that takes the burden off willpower completely.

In Part III, I will give you the Bright Line Eating Food Plan. It is hugely varied because I want to make your weight loss as painless as possible. It's also easily adaptable for any regime you already follow. Whether you are vegetarian, vegan, paleo, gluten-intolerant, have a specific health condition, or need to avoid specific foods, Bright Line Eating will absolutely work for you.

Parts IV and V are about empowering you with tools that make long-term weight loss a sustainable reality. That's the Bright Line Eating difference. We don't tell you what to do and then leave you to figure out how to stick with it over the long term. We are with you every step of the way, for as long as you need us. I have been thin for well over a decade, and I still enjoy the support of this community on a daily basis.

Bright Line Eating ushers in an end to cravings, an end to dieting, an end to that constant, exhausting, soul-sucking loop in your head about food and calories and exercise and pounds. I have no interest in getting you *Thin* if you're not also going to be *Happy* and *Free*. Living Happy, Thin, and Free is your birthright. I do it. My Boot Campers are doing it. And you can, too.

So join me. Join me and the countless others who are walking arm-in-arm on this glorious path. Whatever your background, however much you have or haven't suffered with food, whether you're hundreds of pounds overweight, just a few pounds overweight, or in a right-sized body but crazy with food obsession, we hold the vision of your highest future, your happiest, healthiest, most actualized self. We want you to get Happy, Thin, and Free so that you can be liberated to do what you're here on this earth to do, without being held back by your weight or your relationship with food. You have gifts to give, a purpose to fulfill, and we want you living it.

If I can break free, anyone can. I have no doubt. You've got this.

So. Thank you for letting me share my story.

And now buckle in, because *Bright Line Eating* is about to change your life.

With love,
Susan

Part I

HOW THE BRAIN BLOCKS WEIGHT LOSS

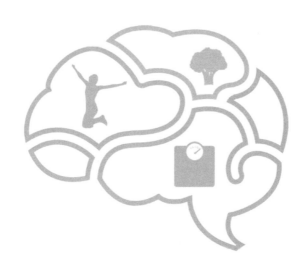

CHAPTER ONE

THE WILLPOWER GAP

So what is happening to those 108 million dieting Americans I mentioned in the Preface? The people unsuccessfully trying to lose weight, some four and five times every year? I posit—and the science supports—that their brains are blocking them from losing weight. "Why?" you might ask. "Why would it *do* that?" It seems contrary to the idea that our bodies can monitor, regulate, and heal themselves. And probably, under normal evolutionary circumstances, they could have. But our modern times have changed many of our behaviors and circumstances. Research shows that modern foods and modern patterns of eating are hijacking three critical processes in our brain and rendering sustainable weight loss nearly impossible. The purpose of Bright Line Eating is to reverse these processes and get the brain back on board with our weight-loss goals. The reason that someone who commits to Bright Line Eating and stays with it loses that excess weight and keeps it off long-term is that, on Bright Line Eating, the brain and the body work in concert with one shared goal: living Happy, Thin, and Free.

Over the next three chapters, I'm going to describe these three critical processes, one at a time; the rest of the book will be devoted to explaining the solution. It's vital that you not just skip this section and jump ahead to the Food Plan because your neighbor already lost 100 pounds and gave you the book and you just want to *do it* already. You need to fully understand what is happening inside your brain—fully understand why Bright Line Eating will work where your other attempts have failed.

In this chapter, I'm going to start by talking about something that most people think they already understand: willpower.

What Is Willpower?

We often think of willpower as an aspect of our moral character, or as a tool that gets more effective with increased commitment. How do we use it? We marshal it. This common phrase reveals our bias—it suggests that all the willpower we need is there, waiting for us to mobilize, rally, raise, and summon it. If we fail to exert the effort, then shame on us.

But willpower isn't what you think it is, and doesn't work how you think it works.

Every January, millions of people in the U.S. start diets. E-mails flood inboxes, ads flood the Internet, every magazine and daytime news show is talking about the latest fad diet and exercise program, and people psych themselves up that *this* time it's going to work. What people don't realize is that these diets are designed to rely on your "willpower" to be effective. They outline what to eat, what not to eat, how to exercise, and why, and then they leave you to manage execution over the long term.

This is why gyms are packed in January and attendance levels fall back to normal in February. This is why, by spring, the average American is already starting his or her *second* diet.

I have asked college students in my classes on introductory psychology and the psychology of eating how they would define willpower. The majority mistakenly believe it's either something in your personality that you're born with or a barometer of inherent moral fiber.

Actually, it's neither.

Willpower is a simple brain function. And while studies have shown that there is a genetic component to how strong it is,[1] there is a lot more to it than genes. It's important to understand that willpower is not merely a mental faculty that resists temptation—it also governs other things, like the ability to focus. It monitors our task performance, regulates our emotions, and, most important, helps us make choices. Have you ever thought to yourself at the end of the day, "I cannot make one more decision!" You tell your spouse or roommate to choose dinner or pick the movie because you just *can't*. That's what scientists call *decision fatigue.*[2] And it's real.

Roy Baumeister is a professor of psychology at Florida State University, and arguably the world's leading expert on willpower, or *ego depletion*, as he calls it. In 1998 he coauthored a paper in the *Journal of Personality and Social Psychology* that put willpower on the map as a subject of scientific inquiry.[3]

In the article he describes what is now famously called The Radish Experiment. Participants were told to fast overnight and arrive hungry at the lab the following morning. They were directed into a room that was filled with the aroma of freshly baked cookies. Then the subjects were asked to sit at a table on which there were two things: a bowl filled with raw radishes, and a plate brimming with chocolate-chip cookies and chocolate candies. One group was told they could eat the radishes while filling out a questionnaire, but were warned not to touch the cookies or candies—they were to be used in another study. A second group was told that they *could* eat the cookies and candies, but to please not touch the radishes. A third group didn't find any food in the room at all. Each participant was given about 15 minutes to complete the questionnaire, then was taken into the adjacent room, where they were told they would "do the actual study." They were led to believe it would be an intelligence test. In reality, it was a set of impossible geometry puzzles. Researchers noted how many attempts the participants would make and how long they would persist in trying to solve them.

The participants who had just resisted the cookies for 15 minutes had little willpower left to force themselves to work on those impossible geometry puzzles. They quit after eight minutes. But participants who were allowed to eat the cookies, and the control subjects who encountered no food at all, persisted in working on those impossible geometry puzzles for nearly 19 minutes, even though they were insolvable. They just kept trying. They had the willpower.

This was the first experiment where researchers realized, "Whoa, willpower is actually a *thing*." Really. Until 1998, scientists didn't know that willpower was measureable. What Baumeister went on to prove is that exerting self-control in one area of our lives uses up this precious, finite resource and prevents further regulation of other functions.[4]

It's vital to understand this, because most of us naturally have only about fifteen minutes of self-regulatory capacity available at a time.* Fifteen minutes. (Can you imagine if your phone only had fifteen minutes of charge?) And a whole host of activities and stressors deplete it, particularly the kinds of things that most of us do all the time, like check e-mail. You may not consciously realize it, but every e-mail you receive requires your brain to make a host of decisions. Delete it? Read it? Store it? Reply? All? Now? Later? How?

Emotional regulation also depletes willpower very quickly. For example: picking your kids up from school, getting them home, through their activities and homework, then dinner, bath time and bedtime, and squabbles and whining, without losing your patience. That depletes willpower, big time. How many times do we want to go straight from turning out our child's bedside lamp to the kitchen? You're not imagining that connection. The link is brain glucose. One study showed that inmates coming up for parole had only a 15 percent chance of getting paroled if

---

* In several studies, a 15-minute exposure to temptation was enough for a large faction of the subjects to have severely impaired performance on a subsequent task.

their parole judge was due for a break—and, presumably, a snack. After the break, their odds went up to 65 percent.[5] How does all this work?

Willpower in the Brain

The seat of willpower in the brain is the **anterior cingulate cortex.**

The anterior cingulate cortex sits right behind the **prefrontal cortex**, which is the seat of rational decision-making in the brain.

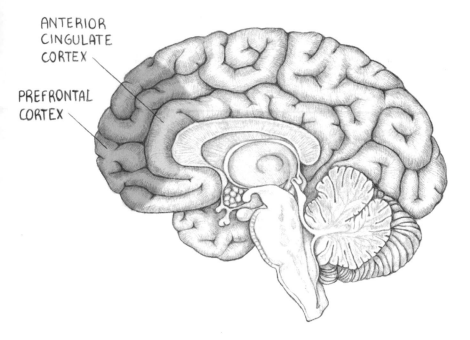

ANTERIOR
CINGULATE
CORTEX

PREFRONTAL
CORTEX

The entire brain runs on glucose, but the anterior cingulate cortex is especially sensitive to glucose fluctuations.[6] When brain glucose levels drop, activity in this area slows to a crawl. The cruelest trick of nature is simply this: after we've been working for a few hours, or at the end of a long day when blood sugar levels are at their lowest, our brains abandon us and leave us incapable of making a wise choice about what to eat.

Which brings us back to our dieters in those first few weeks of January. They start each day with good intentions. They exercise, which depletes their willpower. They have an average day, meaning whether at home with kids, or at work, they are emotionally regulating themselves, which depletes their willpower. They check their e-mail. And they are resisting near-constant temptations to eat. By the time dinner rolls around, many of them will turn to their spouse and say, "Let's just order pizza," and not even know why.

They've just fallen into the Willpower Gap.

How many times have you started the day with great intentions, only to end up ordering takeout for dinner because you were exhausted? You tell yourself, *Oh, well, I'll start again tomorrow.* Or you've been working on a report for a few hours, and then you find doughnuts in the break room? If you eat them, it's not because you're weak. It's because you're normal.

Since resisting temptation is one of the key things that depletes willpower, Roy Baumeister and one of his graduate students wondered how much time people actually spend doing just that. So they decided to find out. With a colleague in Germany, W. Hofmann,[7] they gave subjects beepers and then paged them seven times each day, at random intervals, and asked, "Hey, what are you doing right now? Are you resisting some kind of desire or a craving? If so, what for?" From the 205 male and female participants, they gathered over 7,827 momentary reports. The data were staggering.

People spend, on average, *four hours a day*[8] resisting some kind of desire or craving: sleep, leisure, sex, checking Facebook. These all ranked. But the number-one desire people spent their energy resisting? Food. By far. It's the number-one thing we want. We think about it hours more every day than our brains have the capacity to resist it. It's everywhere, and giving in is socially acceptable (unlike walking out of work to catch a movie or having sex with our cubicle-mate—other popular desires).

Now you're starting to see why the idea that someone could lose weight just by *will*-ing it is pretty ludicrous.

There are things we can do to replenish our stores of will-power. Glucose restores it.[9] Prayer,[10] meditation,[11] social connection,[12] sleep,[13] and gratitude restore it, too.[14] Which is helpful, but scientist Brian Wansink calculated that we make, on average, 221 food-related choices each day.[15] Yes, 221! Even falling into one or two small Willpower Gaps would be enough to create a weight-loss plateau. And most of us are not falling into small Willpower Gaps. We are falling into canyons—the kind that completely derail our weight-loss efforts and send us back to square one. Over, and over, and over again.

Diet programs that focus extensively on how to exercise and what—and what not—to eat, but fail to incorporate a program of behavioral intervention to bridge the Willpower Gap are doomed to be ineffective.

What you need is a plan that assumes you have no will-power at all—because at any given moment you may not—and works anyway. Bright Line Eating is designed to take the burden off willpower. No matter how much you know about nutrition, you'll never succeed if you're making your food choices on the fly. Bridging the Willpower Gap is essential, and that's what Chapter Six is all about. In Chapter Six, I'm going to teach you the techniques that are the bedrock of Bright Line Eating, techniques that helped one of my dearest friends, Pat Reynolds, lose 190 pounds in 14 months—and keep it off.

Most importantly, you'll stop thinking you are weak-willed. You've just been relying on a part of your brain that can't shoulder that kind of responsibility—period. But no worries. We're going to solve that, too.

Case Study: Lynn Coulston

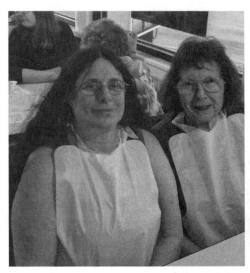 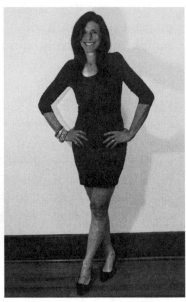

Highest Weight: Over 250 pounds
Current Weight: 103 pounds
Height: 5'2"

It's hard to believe, but I was a really skinny kid. However, for the past 35 years I have gained and lost and gained and lost, tried every diet, and always gained the weight back. I tried the macrobiotic diet, the grapefruit diet, HCG, gallons of SlimFast, gallons of water, Weight Watchers, raw vegan—too many diets, and way too much exercise to remember. Sometimes I got thin. At my lightest, my wedding day, I got down to a size five by starving myself and taking Ex-Lax. I was miserable, but I was thin. I tried to use that same method time and again after that, but I could never get the same results. And the worst part was that it usually took just three weeks after getting thin for me to eat my way back up to, and right past, my previous weight.

Over the following years, I ate whenever I felt emotional stress: from the vending machine at jobs where I felt insecure, as I grieved when my doctor told me that I would never have children, when I was stressed out about school, and when I tried to save my poor mother's life. After her death, I stopped caring about myself completely. At my heaviest, I weighed over 250 pounds. It was at that point that I stopped weighing myself. I cried myself to sleep at night and was always astonished when I woke up still fat. It was as if I thought something would magically remove the pounds. I coped with the disappointment by eating more. I would fill the biggest mixing bowl I have with popcorn, drown it in a bottle of agave syrup, and add lots of salt. Believe it or not, I thought of it as "healthy caramel corn."

My worst food habit was regularly going to Taco Bell for three orders of the taco 12-pack. I would eat one pack all by myself in the car, and then bring the other two home for my husband and me to eat. My husband is 6'1". I finished mine, but he could only eat half a pack at a time!

Eventually, my knees hurt so badly that I couldn't get down the stairs. My husband had to bring food up to me to eat. It was humiliating and painful. I had neuropathy in my toes. I'm sure I was borderline diabetic, but I wouldn't go to the doctor. When I did go out once, for a funeral, I had to leave my skirt unzipped and hope that my fat would hold it up.

Then I became vegan, and eventually I got down to 150 pounds. I was glad, but still perpetually embarrassed by the "apron" of fat around my waist that hung down over my thighs. I thought about my weight all the time, and the despair made me eat foods that would make me start gaining again. I felt completely wrapped up in my food.

Then someone on one of my vegan websites mentioned Bright Line Eating. I watched the introductory videos, and I've never looked back. With Bright Line Eating I lost those last 50 pounds, I'm a comfortable size zero, and I easily fit into my wedding dress. I've been on maintenance for a while now, and am beginning to realize that I can finally trust that I will keep the weight off. Best of all, I feel very relaxed about food since I know exactly what I'm going to eat and know that it will keep me at my goal weight.

I no longer have neuropathy, my body fat is 17 percent, my resting heart rate is 50, my average blood pressure is 90/60, I am on no medication, and I ran a marathon in January. Slowly, but I ran it. Also, I used to be filled with self-loathing and self-doubt. I was chronically depressed. Now I have a completely different and confident self-image, and I'm not at all depressed.

But my biggest reward from Bright Line Eating was freeing my mind up to think about things besides food. There's nothing like knowing that I will always be able to stay at the weight I want. There is a formula, and it works. And it will always work. I am so incredibly grateful for my new way of life!

CHAPTER TWO

INSATIABLE HUNGER

So now, having read Chapter One, you understand that you are not "weak-willed." You are a human being with a human brain. Weakness has nothing to do with it, and programs that rely on your willpower, in the long term, are dooming you to failure. The scientific fact is that limitations arising from the way willpower is wired in the brain, combined with the stressors and pace of our modern world, leave you vulnerable to unhelpful food choices. And those unhelpful food choices set off a cascade of activity in the brain that creates two things: insatiable hunger and overpowering cravings.

That's what we're going to talk about in the next two chapters. Both of these are new phenomena, historically speaking. Hunger is not new, of course. Hunger is a vital human drive that ensures our survival. What's new is that food is ever-available and food is heavily processed, and this turns out to have interesting, and pretty dire, consequences. It warps our natural motivation to eat and morphs it into an entirely new sort of beast.

For the majority of human history, food was scarce. We had to eat *whatever* we could *whenever* we could get it—when it was ripe, or when we had just run fast enough to catch it. We are built to go stretches of time without food because, frequently, we had to. Our bodies quickly adapt to food shortages by lowering our basal metabolic rates and slowing down our functioning to make do with less.[1] In the total absence of food, the body runs on stored glucose for up to three days, and then the liver begins to break down the body's fat stores and muscle tissue so we can keep going.[2] After a few weeks of starvation, the organs themselves start breaking down and turning into fuel. Even during normal weight loss, attempts to burn more calories through vigorous exercise result in a reduced resting metabolic rate.[3] In short, the body is skilled at adapting to survive until food can be found again.

What it's poor at adapting to, it turns out, is a nonstop smorgasbord of calories. And not just any calories—heavily processed and refined calories. Nowhere in our evolution did the human animal have to contend with this. But it's exactly what our modern food systems and patterns of eating provide: an ever-present glut of processed and refined calories. The obesity rates we're seeing are a visual representation of the collective shock our bodies are in from what is being poured into them.

What has this done?

It's broken our brains.

Insatiable Hunger

So what do I mean by *insatiable hunger*? Evolutionarily speaking, it's a new kind of hunger. It's not "Give me fuel to start my day"; it's, "I just ate dinner and a whole bag of chips and now I'm heading to the freezer for ice cream." *Insatiable* hunger.

When I think about it, I remember many times where, as I was ordering dessert after a big meal or heading back to the kitchen for thirds or fourths, I would check in with my body and ask whether it was *hungry*. The resounding response was "no." But my brain quickly shut down that thought because it was irrelevant, threatening even. I *needed* more food. Insatiable hunger had taken over and there was no stopping it.

Scientists have noticed that this urge I remember so vividly differs from real hunger in two key ways. The first unusual thing is that it's accompanied by a strong urge to be sedentary. Think of our modern activities—eating in front of the TV, eating while reading a book, eating while checking e-mail or surfing the web, eating at a sporting event, eating at the movies, eating in our cars. And those aren't even meals! Those are typically between-meal snacks we've sanctioned. We have turned life into a buffet. A continuous, sedentary buffet. I'm making a point of this because we're going to meet a mouse later who's our rodent counterpart.

Now historically, evolutionarily, this was not the case at all. Having fuel on board used to be a biological trigger to get moving. When the berry bushes were heavy and full, and perhaps someone in our tribe had killed a wildebeest, we'd gorge ourselves for a few days and then our brains would tell us to get active. And that was a good thing. It was crucial that we take those calories and use them to ensure our future survival—we had to grow and store more food for the scarce times coming, build some shelter, or go find a mate. Fuel used to result in activity. But now it doesn't. It results in sluggishness.

The second thing that is different about our modern hunger is that eating doesn't actually satiate it. As I wrote in the Introduction, an eating disorder specialist explained to me years ago that overweight subjects report starting to get *hungrier* at the halfway point of a meal. And they typically end the meal *as hungry* as when they started.[4] That is the response of a broken feedback mechanism. To this day, I can completely relate to those findings. I remember when I was obese—I never seemed to get full. Or if I did, it didn't make me want to *not eat*. I was stuffed, uncomfortably full, but I would just wait thirty minutes for the pain to subside and then keep eating.

That isn't how we're supposed to operate. There is a mechanism called compensation that is supposed to govern how we regulate our intake of calories. It will be familiar to any parent who has felt like sometimes their kids will eat anything that isn't locked down, and other times just seem to live on crackers and air. That's compensation. Research shows that if kids have a lot to eat at a meal, they later instinctively decrease intake, almost calorie for calorie.[5] But we are losing that ability.

Professor Brian Wansink, Director of Cornell University's Food and Brand Lab, was curious about the cues we use to determine whether we're full. It should be simple, right? Full should be a feeling. Well, he came up with the ingenious idea of testing that, using self-filling soup bowls. The bowls had hidden hoses attached to the bottom, and for each spoonful the subjects took, the bowls imperceptibly refilled a little.[6] What happened when an empty bowl was no longer available to cue the participants that they "felt full"? They consumed *73 percent more soup* than participants who ate from a normal bowl. Yet, when leaving the lab, both groups gave identical ratings for how full they felt and how much soup they guessed they had eaten. Midway through the experiment, when participants were at the point where they would have emptied one bowlful, had it not been secretly refilling, Brian Wansink asked subjects if they were full. They looked down at the still half-full bowl, and then back up quizzically, replying, "No . . . How could I be? I haven't even finished yet."

What's this about? How did we get here? What's happening to us? Well, it could be a lot of things—a perfect storm of factors. Dr. Alan Goldhamer is the founder of the TrueNorth Health Center and an advocate for plant-based eating. He posits that the increased calorie density of our foods is responsible.[7] Historically, our food didn't have a very high caloric density. We primarily had access to plants, whole grains, and small amounts of animal protein. If we ate a large quantity of vegetables, we still hadn't taken in very many calories. So the receptors in our stomach lining could easily tell the brain how much fuel we had just taken in based on how stretched they were. But now we can eat a doughnut and a drive-through coffee concoction and consume half of our daily caloric needs while barely filling our stomach. Volume of food and calorie consumption are no longer correlated the way they once were.

Another culprit could be artificial sweeteners. I will be talking about them more in Chapter Six, but here are the basics: artificial sweeteners have no calories, so they give the body nothing to burn for fuel, but they actually impact the insulin system in a way very similar to sugar. The sweet flavor hits the tongue, the receptors in the brain light up, and the pancreas floods the bloodstream with insulin so we're all ready to process the bolus of sugar . . . that never comes.[8] That alone can break the feedback loop.

Plus, artificial sweeteners keep us chomping at the bit for something that actually does contain real sugar, and this can result in us overindulging the next time it's available. In 2010, Dr. Terry Davidson and his colleagues in the Department of Psychological Sciences at Purdue University conducted two experiments that showed that rats eating saccharin-flavored yogurt gained about 29 percent more weight than rats eating glucose-flavored yogurt. Replacing sugar with a noncaloric sweetener had the effect of *increasing* their appetite for sweet foods later on, and this resulted in weight gain.[9]

Meals are another factor. Until recently, meals weren't dictated by a personal schedule, they were dictated by a community's schedule. The tribe ate together to make sure that limited resources were distributed fairly. Before the Industrial Revolution, when life revolved around farming, the family fueled up in the morning, paused their work to eat a large meal midday, and then ate again after dark on their way to bed. Once people moved to factories or mines, shift schedules dictated when employees— and sometimes whole towns—ate. Now there is no time of day when it's unacceptable to eat. If a business meeting is before noon, there are Danish pastries on the table; if it's after noon, there's a tray of cookies. There are doughnuts in the break room, bagels and cookies at the PTA meeting. Coffee is everywhere all the time, accompanied by packets of sugar and pots of cream. Every time of day is a time for food. Our children are the biggest victims of this altered mentality. When my girls were very small and I was taking them to classes, I noticed that after every thirty minutes of tumbling or music, goldfish crackers or raisins would be offered. On all of the college and university campuses where I have taught, students have routinely shown up to class with a snack. And in my psychology of eating class, I would always ask for a show of hands: "Who eats breakfast, lunch, and dinner every day, without fail?" The students would stare blankly back at me. We don't eat meals anymore. We graze.

Yes, all of these factors are playing a role. But something much deeper is also going on, and to understand it, we have to look at how hunger is regulated in the brain.

Leptin and the Hypothalamus

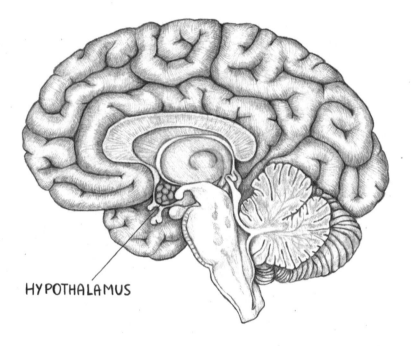

HYPOTHALAMUS

The hypothalamus is an almond-sized area deep inside the brain that contains within it a number of small nuclei with a variety of functions. The hypothalamus is the closest we've got to an internal thermostat. By secreting hormones that in turn stimulate the pituitary gland, it controls hunger as well as body temperature, parenting attachment, sex drive, thirst, fatigue, sleep, and circadian rhythms. It's an important command center, and a lot of vital things are kept in balance here. It's located just above the brain stem, which we'll talk about in a moment.

For now, I want to focus on one hormone in particular and how it affects the hypothalamus's ability to keep our eating in check. That hormone is called leptin.

The story of leptin goes way back to 1949, when a few of the mice in a normal-weight colony grew up to be very, very different than the rest of their littermates.[10] To the astonishment of the scientists, these strange mice weren't active or curious; they didn't dart around the cage like typical rodents. In fact, they almost never moved. Ever. They didn't move . . . but they ate. They just sat by the food trough and ate all day long. And even though all they had to eat were generic pellets, they acted like they couldn't get enough of the stuff. It didn't take long for them to grow to be very, very fat. They loved eating so much that the only way to get those mice to move was to switch the location of the food trough. Then they would waddle, slowly, over to the new location, plop down, and continue to eat. Scientists knew that something important was awry in these special mice, but they couldn't figure out what it was so they kept the strain breeding until the source of the malfunction could be discovered. Finally, in 1994, after working with these unusual, obese mice for eight years, Jeffrey M. Friedman of the Laboratory of Molecular Genetics at Rockefeller University discovered their issue. Way back in 1949, a spontaneous mutation had deprived the mice of a specific recessive mouse gene, the ob gene.[11] Friedman and his colleagues followed the genetic breadcrumbs and discovered what the ob gene does. It makes a specific hormone, and that hormone's job is to signal to the brain that the mouse needs to *stop eating* and to *get active*. Friedman's group called this newly discovered hormone *leptin*, from the Greek word leptos, meaning thin.

Were those mice morally defective? Unintelligent? Lazy? Did they need an educational campaign to teach them to eat moderate amounts of food and get their daily exercise? Nope. They just needed some leptin. It turns out that without leptin, the brain thinks it's perpetually starving. It will never believe it's safe to stop eating and to start to move. It's leptin that says, "Okay! Fueling up is over—go build, go farm, go procreate."

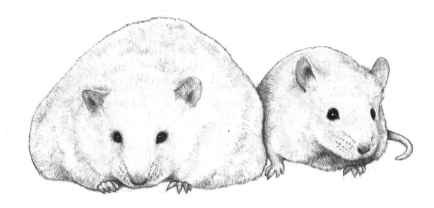

THIS MOUSE IS MISSING
THE GENE THAT MAKES LEPTIN

And sure enough, after they were given a few leptin injections, those mice lost interest in food, started voluntarily climbing into the hamster wheel, and got skinny again.

Eureka!

Of course the pharmaceutical industry immediately threw millions at trying to figure out how to manufacture and patent leptin pills.[12] One little pill, and all of us humans would soon be able to pull ourselves away from the food troughs and jump on the treadmills. Alas, as fate—or biology—would have it, leptin in pill form doesn't make an overweight person lose weight. Nor do direct leptin injections. Why not? Well, we don't have the same problem that those mice did. They were completely missing the gene that makes leptin, so they had no leptin at all. We do. In fact, it turns out that overweight people have even *more* leptin circulating in their blood than skinny people.

This stands to reason, because leptin is produced by fat cells. Leptin is the missing link in our satiety feedback mechanism. When we eat a whole bunch of food, the excess we can't burn immediately goes to our fat cells. As our fat cells get fuller, they secrete more leptin. The leptin circles back up to the brain and says, "No more eating! Go find something useful to do with all this energy."

So why is all this leptin swimming in our blood, but not signaling our brains to tell us we're full? What's causing the breakdown in this finely tuned system? The general answer, which scientists have known for years, is that people are becoming *leptin resistant*.[13] Their brains are not registering, or "seeing," the leptin that's circulating in their blood.

I certainly remember what that felt like. Sitting on the couch night after night, eating, not enjoying it, not even tasting it much of the time, and rarely, if ever, feeling full or satisfied—just equal parts comforted, numb, and disgusted.

So now we ask, what's the underlying cause of leptin resistance? This, my friends, was the holy grail of obesity research. Solve the puzzle of leptin resistance, and you've cracked the code of the obesity pandemic. And not that long ago, it happened. A team at UCSF Medical Center, led by Dr. Robert Lustig, discovered what's causing the widespread epidemic of leptin resistance.

The cause, my friends, is *insulin*. Insulin is blocking leptin in the brain.[14]

Insulin

These days, most of us know a bit about insulin. We know it has something to do with diabetes, and something to do with sugar levels.

And that's a good start.

Here's the deal: Our bodies need blood sugar for energy on a cellular level. However, blood sugar can't go directly into most cells. After you eat and your blood-sugar level rises, the hypothalamus signals the pancreas to release insulin into your bloodstream. Insulin attaches to cells and tells them to open and absorb the blood sugar, which is why it's often called the "key" hormone. Insulin can tell your body to use sugar for energy now, or to store it for future use; it helps keep blood-sugar levels from getting too high (hyperglycemia) or too low (hypoglycemia).

Anyone who has read about the surge of Type 2 diabetes diagnoses in all developed nations knows that the way our global diet has changed is elevating insulin levels far beyond where our bodies were intended to idle. Research on overweight kids has shown that between grade school and high school, baseline insulin levels rise 45 percent.[15] We're talking *average* levels, not the spike that comes from one snack out of a vending machine. The changes in our global diet mean that baseline insulin levels are just too high—in practically all of us.

Scientists knew that obesity was tied to excess insulin, but until the team at UCSF discovered the link between insulin and leptin, we didn't understand what exactly the excess insulin was doing that was so harmful.

But now we know. It's blocking leptin. And in just about the worst place possible, neurologically speaking.

The Brain Stem

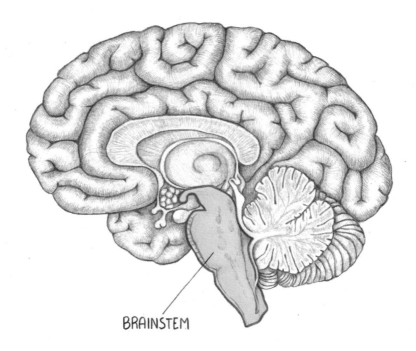

BRAINSTEM

We used to think that leptin was being blocked at the hypothalamus, which is true, and would be bad enough, but now we know that leptin is also being blocked at another place—the brain stem.[16] The brain stem is also sometimes called the "lizard brain." It sits at the base of the brain and is actually structurally contiguous with the spinal cord. Why does it matter that leptin is being blocked at the brain stem? Because this is not one of the parts of the brain that helps us reason, debate, or play out possible scenarios. The brain stem is in charge of the things we *can't* control—basic things like breathing, swallowing, blood pressure, cardiac functions, and whether we're awake or sleepy. In short, there is no overriding the brain stem.

You can try, though, and you might be successful—for a hot second. For example, if you walk briskly up ten flights of stairs, you might "decide" you're only going to take slow breaths through your nose while you're doing it. You could start out that way, but, at some point, your brain stem will take over and demand the oxygen it needs. Like it or not, you will start to breathe heavily. It's not up to you. When it comes to keeping us alive, the brain stem is in charge.

And *this* is where leptin is being blocked! The most primal part of our brain is not getting the hormonal cue that we're full, that we've taken in an adequate amount of food. In those of us with leptin resistance, it is absolutely convinced we are starving. So we sit on the couch as it keeps telling us to eat. And eat. And eat.

And what are we eating? What are we reaching for as a global population?

Exactly the foods that keep our insulin levels elevated in the first place.

Case Study: Linden Morris Delrio

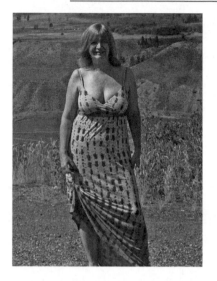 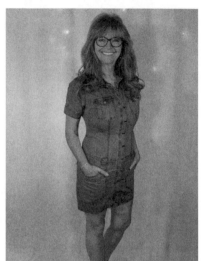

Highest Weight: 189 pounds
Current Weight: 126 pounds
Height: 5'8"

I was born in Edmonton, Alberta, in 1956, the youngest of five children. Our family was quite poor and we didn't have a happy home life. There was a lot of drinking and general dysfunction and I felt psychologically and physically unsafe most of the time. While I struggled to find normalcy, I was also troubled with having to cope with a relatively minor physical defect—I was born missing all four digits on my left hand. I also turned out to be naturally left-handed . . . how crazy is that?

Still I excelled at school at an early age and adapted very well physically. But mentally, I found life pretty hard. I had to endure some amount of teasing and nastiness from other children, and, between the ages of 8 and 11, I was subjected to inappropriate sexual touching. As I reflect, it comes as no small wonder I sought out substances to help me feel better about myself and my circumstances. Food helped to muffle my inner feelings of lack, disgust, and shame. Since we were poor, our food choices were not the healthiest. We ate biscuits smothered in gravy and big bowls of steamed rice soaked in soy sauce for lunch in the dreary, cold prairie winters. I used my church donation money to buy little bags of potato chips on Sundays.

But none of it was ever enough to take away the poverty, addiction, or the dark smudge and stain that I felt life had imprinted upon me.

In junior high school, I discovered that drugs helped my weight management. And so began decade upon decade of struggles to get my weight down—which I did, but only to gain it back again. Worse yet, the general baseline kept rising with each bout.

But I never stopped trying. I was a gym rat, plus did Weight Watchers, Blood Type Diet, Paleo, Atkins, Low-Carb, Low-Fat, No Fat, Dr. McDougall, Dr. Fuhrman, WFPB . . . an endless list really. By 2014 I was thoroughly disheartened and completely disillusioned with myself and with what life seemed to be offering up to me. More than anything, I felt like a fraud and a failure. Sure, I had other successes in my life, but, to be frank, I just couldn't fire on all cylinders with the amount of food I was packing away and the food comas induced by my overconsumption. I actually prayed to become bulimic so I could manage my weight gain. Day after long day, I would wake up planning my food binge for later in the day and would go to sleep at night promising myself that the next day would be different. It never was.

When I discovered Bright Line Eating, I started with a lot of trepidation at first. But with one 24-hour day on the Food Plan under my belt, I was off and running. I was engaged, focused, and committed. I stuck to it, with no deviations, until I reached my goal weight.

In six months I lost a total of 63 pounds and have been easily maintaining a weight between 125–129 for some time now. At 59 years of age, I literally *flew* by my old notions of an ideal weight. I'm now living at a weight I never would have dared dream of!

On most days, my obsession with food has been lifted. I can wear absolutely anything my heart desires and look pretty fantastic in it. I have also overcome a nearly debilitating heart condition, RVOT. I was experiencing potentially fatal heart events on a regular basis, and they have all but gone away.

I have also developed friendships and family here in the Bright Line Eating community that I never thought possible. I never imagined I would receive such care and kindness, much less be in a position to so heartily offer the same to others. My work evolved into my current position as the Director of Online Support Community Services, the very place where I found my own ultimate freedom from the tyranny of my obsession with food.

Slowly, as time passed and I shed pounds, I started taking steps to advance my painting career, and I love my jazz studies in guitar, cello, piano, and voice—an area where I eventually hope to perform at a professional level. Whatever happens, I'm so up for the journey and the awesomeness of day-to-day life.

Everything has changed. I truly feel UNSTOPPABLE most days. I now embody HAPPY, THIN, and FREE and I know if I can do this . . . so can you. Won't you join me?

Viva la Bright Lines!

CHAPTER THREE

OVERPOWERING CRAVINGS

So we've learned that we're eating too much of the wrong foods, the foods that cause our insulin levels to rise. The increased insulin blocks leptin, which makes our brains think we're starving. So we're reaching for *more* food, and our willpower is nowhere in sight because we've used it all up checking e-mail for fifteen minutes. Awesome.

Now that you understand the Willpower Gap and the brain malfunction known as insatiable hunger, we're going to talk about the third way our brains block weight loss—overpowering cravings.

Now, at first glance, "overpowering cravings" may seem very similar to "insatiable hunger." And it's true that the net result of both of them is that we end up eating more food than our bodies need. But they're *not* the same thing.

So what's the difference?

Essentially, they arise from different mechanisms in the brain. Insatiable hunger originates from the fact that leptin is being blocked at the brain stem, which is what drives people to mindlessly put food in their mouths all day, without any ability to get feedback from the body that it doesn't need any more food on board. You might think of this as the "grazing" or "overeating" mechanism. Overpowering cravings, on the other hand, are a "bingeing" mechanism. They are what make people—myself included—drive miles out of their way for that one specific food—their "fix." You can see them late at night in the supermarket, wandering the aisles looking for "that thing" that will "hit the spot." And until they get it, until they can tear open the bag and pop one in their mouth or sit in the parking lot of the supermarket shoveling food in because they can't stand to wait through the drive home, until they know that release is imminent, their entire body is rigidly focused on one thing: scratching that itch in their brain.

But where does that itch originate?

The Nucleus Accumbens

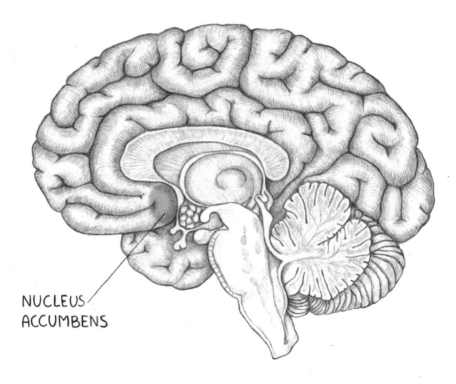

NUCLEUS
ACCUMBENS

The nucleus accumbens is the seat of pleasure, reward, and motivation in the brain. Inside its outer shell is a cluster of neurons that are activated by dopamine and designed to motivate our behavior, which is why so many life-sustaining activities stimulate the brain to release dopamine—sex, exercise, and yes, eating.

In thinking about what's going on in our nucleus accumbens every day, I want to talk specifically about two things: food and sex. We may not generally think of them as being linked, but they're both essential. In order for our species to survive, we have been primed to respond to certain sexual and edible stimuli—sights and smells—with, essentially, "I want to get me some of that." Interestingly, those stimuli have changed over the years in parallel ways. We simply do not have equivalent food and sexual stimulation available to us as we had 100,000 years ago, or 1,000 years ago, or even 50 years ago.

Let's just stay on sex for a moment. If we think about the kind of sexual stimuli that existed a long time ago, we're talking about getting glimpses. If you were lucky and you stumbled upon a river where people from the next community over were bathing, you might catch sight of a naked body at an angle, but you'd be hiding, not that close, and your view would be obscured. In short, you wouldn't have access to much stimulation on call, anytime you wanted it. In contrast, the pornography that's available today 24/7 on the Internet is grotesquely intense.

The brain is no match for that kind of stimuli, for the amount of dopamine that it releases. The brain simply wasn't designed to process a chemical flood of that magnitude. When you start pumping that much dopamine into the nucleus accumbens, it responds by essentially saying, "Whoa, that is *really excessive*. We don't need anywhere near that kind of stimuli around here." If you do that over and over again, it adapts by downregulating.

Downregulation

Downregulation is the process whereby the brain thins out dopamine receptors to adapt to the overload. The next time a similar onslaught comes, its response can be more appropriate.

That sounds great, except that now you're changing the physiology of the brain. If the stimulation is not forthcoming, you don't feel very good.

What's that like?

As a former crystal meth and crack cocaine addict—two substances that practically wipe out the dopamine receptors in the nucleus accumbens—I feel qualified to weigh in here a bit. And what I'll say is this: using drugs didn't feel pleasurable. Maybe at first, but not after a while.

What did it feel like?

It felt like "*More.*"

I just wanted more.

But once the dopamine downregulation kicked in, the state I was left in between fixes absolutely felt like the *absence* of pleasure. Completely and totally bleak. It felt itchy. It felt needy. It felt not okay, and I would have to go get more to escape. Not to get high, but to get *normal*. This is something I think a lot of people misunderstand. They think the addict is using to get high, but really the addict is using to get normal. To just be okay for a bit.

When we look at food, it's the exact same story. If you think about the availability and intensity of sweet foods 100,000, or 1,000, or 50 years ago compared with today, the difference is striking. Take 100,000 years ago: you were lucky when the berry bushes were in season or you could safely get some honey away from the bees. Today, berries are the foods people tell you to eat when you're trying to quit sweets.

Refined sugar didn't enter our diets until the 1700s. It was difficult to access and to process prior to that, so it was reserved for nobility or people of means. With the advent of the sugar plantation, all that changed. After World War II, we started mechanizing food production. Food became a corporate product with large marketing forces behind it. Then, in 1973, a massive change in U.S. farming subsidy policy brought high-fructose corn syrup onto the scene as an inexpensive sweetener, and consumption increased again. But whether we're talking about high-fructose corn syrup, good old fashioned table sugar, or any of the dozens of sugars clothed in other names, the reality is that 80 percent of the calories sold on supermarket shelves are laced with it.[1] It tastes good, and it makes our brain *feel* good. As a result, over just the last few decades, sugar consumption has skyrocketed to ridiculous levels, and that means that we are hitting the brain with ever-higher, more potent levels of stimulation. Stimulation it simply wasn't designed to handle.

Cravings

So that is what's happening in the brain. We are flooding its receptors with dopamine and they are thinning out. How often does this really happen? Well, think about everything we covered in Chapter Two—leptin is being blocked in our brain, so we keep going back for more and more food. If someone is eating processed foods at every meal, or even more often, those dopamine receptors are being hit with excessive stimulation every few hours or more.

And, of course, there are many other types of stimulation in our modern lives that flood the brain with excess dopamine: drinking coffee all day, smoking cigarettes, regularly watching pornography, using cocaine or amphetamines, and drinking alcohol. But honestly, just eating a lot of sugar and flour will do it.

Yup. When it comes to food, those are the two culprits. Sugar and flour.

In fact, I want you to consider looking at sugar and flour in an entirely new way. People tend to think of sugar and flour as *foods*.

I invite you to start looking at them as *drugs*.

Sugar and Flour in the Brain

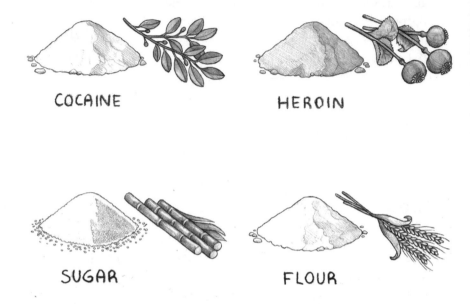

COCAINE

HEROIN

SUGAR

FLOUR

These drawings are renditions of photographs taken from the web. I highly recommend you do a Google image search for these same substances so you can see with your own eyes what I'm about to describe. For obvious reasons, I couldn't commission photographs of heroin and cocaine to show you, but it's worth seeing how eerily alike all these substances look. The upper left corner depicts cocaine. Cocaine, we all agree, is a drug. But how does it *become* a drug? Where does it come from?

Cocaine is derived from the coca leaf, which grows in Colombia and other regions of South America. On their own, coca leaves are pretty harmless. Hikers in the Andes Mountains chew on them all the time. What happens when you put a coca leaf inside your cheek and chew on it? Your cheek gets a little numb and you get a little lift, like drinking half a cup of caffeinated tea.

Does the pleasure you get from that make you break into your grandmother's house to steal her DVD player so you can buy more coca leaves? No, it doesn't. Coca leaves are not addictive.[2] But when you take the *inner essence* of those coca leaves and refine and purify that inner essence into a fine powder . . . you now have a drug.[3] A very powerful drug. Cocaine.

In the upper right corner, we have heroin. Heroin comes from the poppy plant. What happens if you sit in a field and eat poppy plants all day long? You'll fail a urine test for opium, but you're not going to become addicted. You're not going to become an itching, shriveling heroin addict. It's only when you take the *inner essence* of that poppy plant and refine and purify it into a light-brown powder that you get the drug called heroin.

Next comes sugar. Where do we get sugar? From the sugarcane plant, sugar beets, and corn. These are all foods that I myself would eat freely. Sugarcane is hard to come by in the Northeast so I've never actually nibbled on it, but I eat beets on my salad most nights. I love corn on the cob. In fact, just a ways up from my house there is a farm stand that sells fresh corn on the cob all summer. Yum. Not addictive—healthy. But when you take the inner essence of those plants and you refine and purify it into a powder (or, in the case of high-fructose corn syrup, a thick liquid), now you have a drug. You've taken a food and you've turned it into a drug.

And finally, flour. Where do we get flour? Well, from any number of plants. They all start as healthy foods—in their whole form. But when you take their inner essence and you refine and purify them into a fine powdery substance, you now have a drug.

If, as you read this, you feel bleak and desperate at the thought of going without sugar and flour, I just want to point out that *that*, right there, is dopamine downregulation talking. It's amazing how powerful the feeling can be—we think that, if these foods aren't in our life, then there is nothing good to live for. I know what that feeling of bleakness is like. You'll get through it, I promise. Dopamine receptors do regenerate. You will be fine. You'll be *better* than fine, because soon enough you'll be well on your way to your goal weight, much happier, much more confident, and free from the damage these substances are inflicting on your brain.

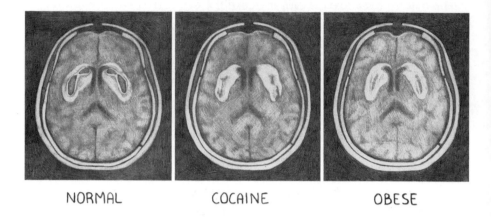

NORMAL   COCAINE   OBESE

Here we have an artist's rendition of three PET scans of different brains and their dopamine responses in the nucleus accumbens. On the left is a normal brain exhibiting a healthy dopamine response, as represented by the darker shading—the darker the shading, the stronger the neurological activity. In the center is a scan of a brain addicted to cocaine. Note that the response is pretty muted. But look—on the right is the brain of an obese person. See how little dark shading there is? The dopamine response is actually worse than the cocaine addict's.

Now, one of the guiding principles in science is "correlation doesn't prove causation." In other words, it's possible that, instead of overeating *causing* the thinning out of the dopamine receptors, it could have been the reverse. Perhaps the obese brain demands so much food because it was born without enough dopamine receptors in the first place.

Scientists continued to entertain this possibility until May of 2010, when a Scripps Research Institute paper was published in *Nature Neuroscience*.[4] Dr. Paul Johnson and Dr. Paul Kenny took rats with normal, healthy brains and split them up into three groups. The control group was fed standard laboratory rat pellets. The second group was fed a diet of bacon, sausage, cheesecake, pound cake, frosting, and chocolate, but only for one hour each day. The third group got access to that diet for 18 to 23 hours a day—all they could eat—a rat buffet. No surprise, the third group got really obese. But, more important, they started with healthy brains and ended with downregulation in their dopamine receptors. The diet *caused* their brains to change.

Science had finally proven what anyone who has ever been in a 12-Step program for food already knows: food addiction is real. As real as cocaine addiction. As real as heroin addiction. There is no physiological difference. Initially, researchers asked, "Really? Food is as addictive as cocaine and heroin?" But now, a lot of researchers estimate that it might be *more* addictive.

Sugar and Flour Addiction

In 2007 at the University of Bordeaux, Dr. Serge H. Ahmed's team injected rats with intravenous cocaine until they were addicted. Then the team offered them something they had never been exposed to before: sweetened water. The rats were forced to make a choice between the intravenous cocaine they were already addicted to and sweetened water. It made no difference whether the sweetener was sugar or saccharine—those rats preferred the sweetened water.[5] Based on that study, Dr. Mark Hyman estimates that sugar is *eight times* more addictive than cocaine.[6]

In the Scripps Research Institute study, rodents would willingly cross and stand on an electrified floor in order to keep eating their high-sugar food. You can measure the strength of an addiction by titrating the strength of the shock that a subject will voluntarily withstand to keep consuming the substance.[7] And the rats' levels went right up to the cocaine- and heroin-addiction thresholds.

Another thing worth noting is that when the researchers took away this hyperpalatable "food" and left the rats with standard rat chow, they starved themselves. They were not interested in eating anything other than the processed, highly rewarding foods. The researchers called this the "salad bar option," and the rats wanted no part of it.[8]

So how do we know which foods are addictive? Some popular researchers and authors have suggested that the addictive elements are sugar, fat, and salt.[9] I don't agree with all three of these. First of all, to my knowledge, there is no evidence that salt is addictive. True, salt makes food more *palatable*, leading to the consumption of more calories. In one study, people consumed 11 percent more food if it was pleasantly salted.[10] But *palatable* is not the same as *addictive*.

How about fat? Well, here the research is trickier, especially since most high-fat foods also contain sugar, flour, or both. But in 2013, the landscape finally became clear. Three scientists conducted an ingenious study that pitted fat directly against sugar and watched what happened in the brains of the people who consumed different quantities of each.

Researchers put subjects in an fMRI machine and measured the activity in various parts of the brain as they sucked chocolate milkshakes through straws. The levels of sugar versus fat in the milkshakes were titrated to create four versions: high sugar/high fat, high sugar/low fat, low sugar/high fat, and low sugar/low fat.[11] The results showed that it was sugar content, not fat content, that drove the response in the reward centers of the brain. For me, this study went a long way toward putting the idea that fat is addictive to bed. Just like salt, fat helps make foods more palatable, and will certainly drive the passive overconsumption of calories, but that doesn't mean it's addictive.

For those of you who are still not convinced, let me put it another way. If you put butter and salt on broccoli, people will eat a bit more broccoli because it tastes better. But I think we all know no one is going to get rich opening salted, buttered broccoli drive-throughs.

Another way to get clear data on this is to just ask people, as I have asked students in my psychology of eating classes, "What foods do you drive out of your way to go buy?" The answers? Cake, cupcakes, cookies, candy, ice cream, doughnuts, chocolate, pizza, chips, pasta, bagels, bread, crackers, and pancakes.

Pizza, chocolate, and chips are the top three most addictive foods.[12] Why is pizza so addictive? Well, let's think about it. Pizza is made out of dough, sauce, and cheese. Sauce is yummy. And cheese can be a little addictive. There are casomorphins in cheese, which mimic an opioid response in the brain. But what happens if you put cheese and sauce on broccoli? You have a delicious side dish for your dinner, but nothing worth venturing out for in a snowstorm. It's the *flour* that's driving the addictive response in pizza. In fact, notice that two of the top three most addictive foods—pizza and chips—are flour-based.

If you want to get Happy, Thin, and Free, it's crucial to be clear about what the addictive foods are because with addiction, "one is too many, and a thousand never enough." Other foods are fine in moderate amounts. Fat and salt can be included in your daily diet in moderate quantities because, without sugar and flour in the mix, they aren't going to derail your efforts. But add sugar or flour to the equation and it's game over.

The Downregulated Life

Dr. Robert Lustig of UCSF, one of the leading experts on sugar in the United States, posits that it takes only three weeks of regular overstimulation for addiction to take hold and the receptors in our brain to thin out.[13] And once those receptors downregulate, several things happen. First, as I said before, life in between eating feels bleak, which is one of the links between the Standard American Diet and depression. Second, the ability to taste food actually diminishes.[14] Not only that, studies have shown that the anticipatory expectation of food in the brain of an obese person is much greater than in a slender person's, but when they eat, the pleasure they derive from the meal is *lower*.[15] In other words, if you're on one of those diets we discussed in Chapter One, and you start to think about how amazing it would be to eat something off your plan, your brain is exaggerating the payoff that that food is going to deliver. But when you actually eat, the payoff won't come. You'll just be left craving the next hit.

I used to live like that—late nights scavenging the supermarket aisles for cookie-dough ingredients, pints of ice cream, bags of chips, and boxes of pasta. I'd go home and eat compulsively, waiting for some feeling—a feeling of being *done*—that never came. I would finish. Finish the whole bowl, the bag, the pint—but I was never done.

Until I was done with sugar and flour completely.

Case Study: Dennis Fansler

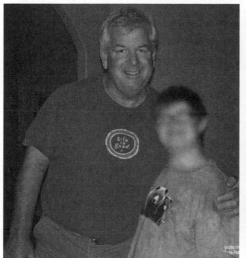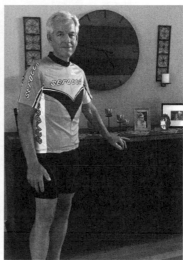

Highest Weight: 280 pounds
Current Weight: 181 pounds
Height: 6'0"

I grew up eating the Standard American Diet: lots of meat and pota-toes, lots of sweets. Add to that life's stressors and a few years ago I topped out at 280 pounds. I felt so depressed and isolated. For 35 years, I had been trying to control my relationship with food, but after so many failed attempts I thought it was just hopeless. Then, after a bad heart scan indicated some blockage in my coronary arter-ies, I got so scared I lost 50 pounds over the next six months. But, as was common for me, I quickly started to gain it back.

Then I came across Bright Line Eating. I was impressed by Susan Peirce Thompson's story and the information she shared in the *Food Freedom* video series. I committed to the plan and my weight dropped off really quickly. I lost 35 pounds in the first 70 days and got down to a weight that's lower than my college football days— when I had about 10 percent body fat. My waist went from about 40 inches to 32. My blood pressure went from 120/80 to 100/60 and my cholesterol went from 237 on 20 milligrams daily of Lipitor to 160, with no medication needed.

But more than that, I appreciate the structure and support I have found in Bright Line Eating. I know that, while I'm happier and less stressed, I need to keep working on the inner change, and Bright Line Eating gives me a space and framework to do that. The greatest change is my newfound belief that I can stay in this new body and spend my time helping others instead of obsessing over food. Bright Line Eating worked for me when nothing in the last 35 years ever had. I tell people, "Be prepared to change your *life,* not just your body size." Anything short of total change is a waste of time.

CHAPTER FOUR

THE SUSCEPTIBILITY SCALE

So now we understand the three ways the brain blocks weight loss. And everyone is equally exposed. We're all saddled with the Willpower Gap because we all have an anterior cingulate cortex that gets fatigued by checking e-mail and holding our tongues. And we all have opportunities throughout the day to fall prey to the Willpower Gap because we're confronted with sugar and flour everywhere we turn.

Given all this, the next natural question that arises is, "Why isn't *everyone* obese?"

It's a very legitimate question.

And I have an answer for you.

Essentially, everyone's equally *exposed*, but not everyone is equally *susceptible*.

Let me explain. A lot of people think that addiction has to do with the substance—that heroin is inherently addictive, and therefore anyone who uses heroin for any extended period of time will, by definition, get hooked. If you're defining addiction in terms of tolerance and withdrawal, then maybe so. Yet if we send 100,000 people home after surgery with several weeks' supply of Vicodin, what we'll find is that some won't take it at all, others will wean themselves off easily despite the withdrawal symptoms, and some will become truly addicted. Alcohol is both addictive and widely used, but we all know that not everyone becomes an alcoholic. Some people can be on-and-off-again smokers, or drink caffeine only when they want some. In essence, some people can take it or leave it.

And some people just can't.[1]

When it comes to sugar and flour, I erroneously assumed for many years that either you *are* a food addict or you *are not.* Certainly in food addiction recovery programs, the first step is to decide whether or not you're powerless over food. But when I looked at the problem as a scientist, I started to see a more nuanced picture emerge. Human traits tend to fall on a bell curve. Why shouldn't addictive susceptibility follow this pattern as well? This wasn't idle intellectual curiosity. The more I applied this idea to the people I was working with, the more it became clear that I was on to something. There were lots and lots of people who clearly weren't food addicts to the degree that I was, and they weren't about to go get help from a 12-Step food addiction program like I had used because they truly didn't belong there. Yet they were addicted to food to some degree, most definitely had a weight problem, and knew the usual diets were never going to work for them. I came to believe that, in order for them to get truly Happy, Thin, and Free, they would first have to understand how susceptible *their* brains were, and then proceed from there.

And that's why I created the Susceptibility Scale.

The Susceptibility Scale ranges from 1 on the low end to 10 on the high end, and it helps you understand how strongly your brain reacts to the reward value of addictive foods.

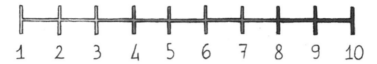

When I began to develop this idea, my e-mail list had several hundred subscribers, and I was writing about the Susceptibility Scale regularly. People wrote in, asking if I had a quiz or an instrument that would tell them how susceptible they were. Creating just such an instrument became one of my top priorities.

So I developed the Susceptibility Quiz, also known as the Food Freedom Quiz. It's only five questions, but they target exactly the dimensions that differentiate people for whom food is not an issue from people who battle its addictive pull. The quiz is framed to analyze your relationship with food during your *worst three months* of eating behaviors. Why? Because once you've engaged in behaviors like regular binge eating, those fiber tracts are laid in the brain. They might not be *active* anymore, but they never go away, so you'll always have to be more vigilant around food than someone who has never struggled in that way.

Are you curious to know how you score? The questions are simple, but the scoring is actually quite complicated, so I've set up a quiz online to calculate it all for you. You can go right now to www.FoodFreedomQuiz.com and find out your Susceptibility Score. I'll explain your results to you when you get back. Go ahead. It will just take you a couple of minutes. I'll wait.

Results

1–3: Low Susceptibility

In our ancient, evolutionary past, low susceptibility probably wouldn't have conferred a survival advantage, but in today's obscenely abundant food environment, you can consider yourself lucky. Your body gives you reliable signals about when to stop eating. In fact, if you're among the lowest of the low, you may even have the problem of not thinking about food *enough*. If you're engaged in a busy day, you might actually forget to eat and have to organize your life to remember to eat the right foods at the right times.

When *The Curious Case of Benjamin Button* came out, Brad Pitt and Cate Blanchett were on *Oprah*, and a fan who happened to be a chef offered to cook them their favorite foods. She asked what they most loved to eat. Both movie stars sat there, stumped. After several awkward moments, the best Cate Blanchett could muster was, "A bowl of rice is nice sometimes." Brad Pitt chimed in with, "Yeah, food's not really on my radar screen." I was floored. How could they *not know* what they most loved to eat? This was *so* not my experience. Oprah leaned out to the audience and declared, "I don't know about you all, but I could NEVER say what those two just said!" Everyone laughed, and the tension was broken. But if you're low on the Susceptibility Scale, that's what your relationship to food is like. Food is simply fuel, of no particular interest at all, or it's a momentary pleasure that quickly passes and is then forgotten.

So, if you score in the 1–3 range, can Bright Line Eating still be helpful? Actually yes, it can.

One of my online Boot Campers, Darlene Saeva, was a serious runner. She trained regularly, and had run 28 marathons during her adult years. But then, in 2013, she had a serious upper-cervical neck injury and was forced to stop running. Despite the fact that she had always been a careful eater, within a year she had gained 28 pounds. Not a huge amount of weight, but it bothered her. She knew a lot about nutrition and tried multiple diets, but none provided enough guidance on exactly *what* and *how much* to eat, so she stayed heavy. Finally, someone told her about the Bright Line Eating Boot Camp, and she signed up. She lost her excess 28 pounds quite rapidly, is now living happily at goal weight, and continues to do Bright Line Eating to this day. Despite the fact that she is only a 2 on the Susceptibility Scale, she loves the structure that Bright Line Eating provides and the clarity that it brings to her eating. She finds that, so long as she sticks with the plan, she stays easily and exactly at her goal weight. If she deviates, she momentarily gains a couple of pounds. But since she's low on the scale and doesn't much care about food, sticking with it is super easy. Hence, she *loves* Bright Line Eating and is delighted that it's solved her weight problem.

Surprisingly, many people who are overweight or even obese are low on the Susceptibility Scale. The combination of a slow-to-normal metabolism coupled with mindless consumption of the quickest, cheapest, most palatable foods around will pack on the pounds, addiction or no. And if getting that weight off becomes a paramount concern, Bright Line Eating can easily come to the rescue. Other people who are low on the Susceptibility Scale seek out Bright Line Eating simply because they want to be the best version of themselves, eating whole foods and living in a body with a balanced insulin system that has consistent energy for all of life's adventures. For people on the low end of the scale, it's a choice, not a necessity.

4–7: Midrange Susceptibility

If you're in the midrange, you may think of yourself as being somewhat challenged by food. How challenged probably depends on whether you're overweight and whether or not you have health issues. But you're no stranger to cravings. Given the hyperpalatable foods that exist today and their near-constant availability, midrange people are in danger of becoming overweight just by eating too much of the wrong foods—or even too much of seemingly healthy foods! I recently had a woman in my Boot Camp who was a plant-based eater, and very health conscious. But before the Boot Camp she was eating too much flour, which was making her sedentary, depressed, and frustrated—because she thought she was doing everything "right." Now she has finally lost the 40 pounds that plagued her for years and is full of energy. About 24 percent of the people who sign up for the Bright Line Eating Boot Camp are in the midrange on the Susceptibility Scale, and they tend to get fabulous results. When you've experienced cravings, stubborn weight gain, and persistent overeating despite a desire to get trim and healthy, finally getting Happy, Thin, and Free is a huge relief.

My mother is also in the midrange on the Susceptibility Scale; she's done the Boot Camp and is a Bright Lifer. I know her relationship with food almost as well as I know my own. When she deviates from the Bright Lines, it's not devastatingly painful and all-consuming, like it is for me. And she finds it much easier to get back on track. But, over the years, she's discovered that there's a very strong correlation between how free she feels and how faithfully she sticks to her Bright Lines. She embraces the Bright Lines because they give her full and complete liberation from any mental chatter about her food, and because she loves having her food *handled* and, of course, living effortlessly in a right-sized body.

8–10: High Susceptibility

If you're highly susceptible, you've probably struggled with your eating and/or your weight for years, if not decades. The signals that tell other people to stop eating just don't work reliably, and it's possible they never did. You might be a "foodie" with cookbooks lining the shelves, or you might not care at all about the fanciness of the food you eat and just spend your mornings thinking about your coffee and doughnut. Or three.

On the Susceptibility Scale, I am a perfect 10. There are many times in life when it's great to be a "Perfect 10." This isn't one of them. In fact, to quote *This Is Spinal Tap*, I probably go all the way to 11.

What does that mean? It means that I can't count points. I can't have a "splurge day" or even a "splurge hour." (I'm looking at you, Carbohydrate Addict's Diet.) I can't eat a slice of pizza on Sunday and go back to salad on Monday. And if I *do* have a slice of pizza, I want many more. Then I go hunting around for some cookies or chips or ice cream to wash it all down. I have been known to rearrange a whole day so I could drive way across town to satisfy a specific food craving. Eating past the point of fullness was a common occurrence. And all of this bothered me. A lot. I thought about it way more than I wished I did, and tried ad nauseam to get my food choices and my weight under control. At times I'd feel like a certain plan or approach was working for me, but those periods never lasted, and before long the struggle would be back. Essentially, my brain is wired to ensure that I would fail at every diet I ever tried. Only the Bright Line Eating approach worked for me.

Here's the simple truth. Plans based on moderation DO NOT work for people who are high on the Susceptibility Scale.

A word about the developers of diet and health-related programs. By and large, they tend to be in the low to midrange on the Susceptibility Scale. Since they are not overly susceptible to the pull of addictive foods, they are able to "solve" their weight problem with diet and/or exercise (or maybe they never even had a weight problem at all). Then they write a book about their success and sell their plan as a solution that will work for the masses. Well, if you're high on the Susceptibility Scale, like I am, then you and I both know it won't. Because we've tried them all. And nothing worked.

Whether you do Bright Line Eating or not, I want you to become a savvy consumer of diet and exercise programs. When you're presented with a new plan, I want you to ask yourself, *"Where is the creator of this program on the Susceptibility Scale?"* and then look for clues in his or her story to answer that question. If it's a plan designed by someone whose Susceptibility Score appears to be lower than yours, odds are that the solution they're peddling isn't going to be potent enough for the way your brain is wired.

Skinny Highs and Big Lows

If you've taken the quiz and your results surprised you because of your appearance, please do not assume that just because you are slim you will be low on the scale, or just because you are heavy you will be high on the scale. Yes, susceptibility is correlated with weight, but, as you can see from this table,* not nearly as highly correlated as you might expect. In fact, a full 22 percent of people at a normal weight are high on the Susceptibility Scale.

BMI Category	Low Susceptibility	Midrange Susceptibility	High Susceptibility	Total
Underweight	26%	27%	47%	100%
Normal Weight	34%	44%	22%	100%
Overweight	32%	43%	25%	100%
Obese	19%	48%	33%	100%
Very Obese	12%	32%	56%	100%

---

* Because our message is about weight loss and food addiction, the people who come to our website and take the quiz will never be a representative sample of the population. So, to get a fair cross-section of respondents, we hired an independent research company to collect data from a representative sample of 1,300 adults from across the United States.

In my psychology of eating class, I used to draw a big circle on the board and tell my students, "This represents your actions, your attention, your life—the sum total of every thought you have, everything you do, and everything that matters to you." Then I would ask, "What proportion is taken up by thinking about what you've eaten or not eaten, whether you've exercised or not, whether you're on your food plan or off?" And semester after semester, I'd have slender students whisper in shame and horror, "95 percent."

Where does this come into play? These frequently are the people who, twenty years later, will enter my Boot Camp saying, "I don't understand what's happened. I was always thin." Thin *until.* Until they took a sedentary job, gave up sports, got pregnant, or went through menopause. On average, American adults gain five pounds every holiday season[2] and don't lose them. Those pounds add up.

A slender person who is high on the Susceptibility Scale and who doesn't have any resources may run into trouble with their weight at some point. Or, they may not. They may just spend their life as a skinny person restricting, bingeing, purging, over-exercising, abusing laxatives, counting calories, and obsessing over every morsel of food and every pound of weight. Their quality of life will be diminished *every single day* as they suffer quietly with a problem that doesn't make sense and that they think no one understands. They struggle; they just don't wear the evidence on their bodies.

On the other end of the spectrum are people who are overweight but low on the Susceptibility Scale. And here's the thing: people forget that addictive substances have heightened reward salience *even for people who are not addicted.* In other words, sugar and flour taste good and feel good. Every brain loves that nice rush of dopamine, so even if there's no downregulation in the mix, sugar and flour can easily trick you into eating too much of them. This is how, in our current society, people who are in the low or midrange on the Susceptibility Scale so easily become overweight. Foods made mainly out of flour and sugar are readily available, easy to grab, and screaming to be put in our mouths. Before long, our baseline level of insulin has risen and our leptin is being blocked. So our brains think we're starving and we unwittingly eat more and more. In modern-day life, it's becoming the average natural state.

The Data

We have a large and rapidly growing Bright Line Eating community, and we occasionally run campaigns to educate people about their Susceptibility Score and what it means for their life. Over 350,000 people have taken the quiz so far.

It's important to keep in mind that this is anything but a representative sample of the overall population. People, by and large, are drawn to Bright Line Eating because they are unhappy with their weight, their relationship with food, or both. Of course it makes sense that the distribution of respondents would be heavily skewed toward the high end of the scale. So my team and I decided to find out what the breakdown is in the U.S. population at large. Representative samples of the entire population are exceedingly hard to come by, but there are research companies who perform surveys just like this, and do it well, so we hired one of them to find out for us. Here are the data:

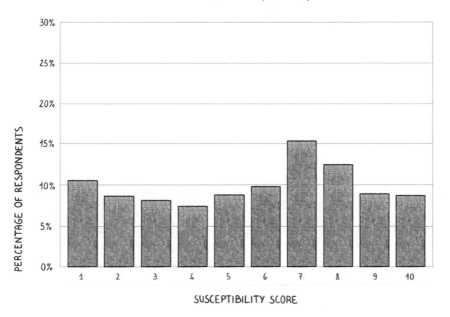

Distribution of susceptibility scores

As you can see, the scores are relatively even, with a slight hump in the 7–8 range. Roughly speaking, one-third of people fall into the low range, one-third are in the midrange, and one-third are high, with around 18 percent of people in the very high (9–10) range, which mirrors research from Yale showing that roughly 19 percent of the population are food addicts.[3] This is very interesting, because we have rat data on addictive susceptibility and, curiously enough, rats are just like us. One-third are highly susceptible to addiction, one-third are moderately susceptible, and one-third are just not susceptible at all.[4] That non-susceptible third just doesn't care too much about the intravenous cocaine. Once it's gone, they're not hunting around for more. They behave like they're thinking, "Okay, that was nice, but I don't miss it." They might be the Brad Pitt and Cate Blanchett of rodents.

Goal Trackers vs. Sign Trackers

I want to go a bit in-depth here about how scientists discovered that one-third of rats are prone to addiction and one-third are not. This research gives us a window into what it is that makes someone susceptible to addiction in the first place. What exactly is it in our environment that triggers such vulnerability in some of us? It's an important question that yields some truly empowering answers.

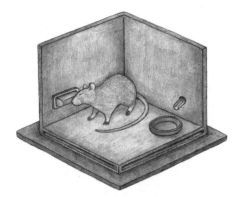

SIGN TRACKER
(ADDICTABLE)

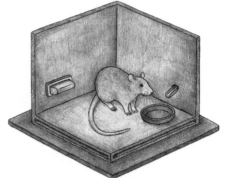

GOAL TRACKER
(NON-ADDICTABLE)

In 2006, at the University of Michigan's Molecular and Behavioral Neuroscience Institute, Shelly Flagel performed some telling rat experiments.[5] She and her team placed rats in standard cages that included a simple retractable lever and a food dish. At random times, the lever would suddenly pop into the cage, and it would stay there for eight seconds. At the end of the eight seconds, the lever was retracted and a food pellet was delivered to the dish. The rats quickly associated the arrival of the lever with the arrival of food. That's straightforward because we are all, rats and humans alike, fast at identifying the cues that tell us food is coming—the smell of bacon, the sound of plates being put on the table before dinner, the sight of a meal coming together on the stove—across all of our senses, there are cues that make us salivate.

What electrified the researchers is what happened next. When the lever appeared, some rats immediately ran to the dish and waited for the food to arrive. These were the "goal-tracking" rats, and their behavior was expected. They were pulled toward the goal: the food. But other rats, lots of them, ran over to the lever instead! Not the life-sustaining food. Nope. They loved the lever. The cold, metal lever, which provided no tangible benefit to them whatsoever. They nuzzled it. They sniffed it. They scampered around it. They couldn't eat or drink it, yet their brains quickly adapted to tracking for it—and released dopamine when they saw it. Their lives quickly became oriented around the lever. The researchers called these rats "sign trackers" because they were pulled in by the sign, the cue, that was associated with food.

What This Means for Us: Eating, Cues, and Emotions

You might be thinking, "But I don't have a lever come into my kitchen before I cook. How does this apply to me?" Well, if you are a human being who is powerfully attracted to the cues that predict food rewards in our society, then life might go something like this . . .

You're walking in a mall and suddenly you're drawn down a corridor and don't even know why, because you didn't even register seeing the Cinnabon sign out of the corner of your eye. But you did. Your brain picked up on a cue that predicts reward. Or you're a teacher and you're just walking past the lounge when you get a glimpse of a pink box through the window and, before you know it, you're "deciding" to go talk to a colleague you see in there. And, of course, eat a doughnut. Or two. Our highways are one long path strung with reward cues: golden arches, a purple bell, a giant ice cream cone. We are inundated with visual reward cues.

But visual cues aren't the only cues. Time of day is also a powerful cue. If you always drive to a Starbucks to get a pick-me-up on the way home, you are cued to want caffeine at that time of day. Or, when you've finally gotten your kids down, that means it's time to go sit on the couch and have your reward. This is a very common one, and closely tied to the Willpower Gap— think about how much willpower was depleted just getting you to that moment.

In fact, the Willpower Gap comes into play across the board, because even if you are vigilant 95 percent of the time, there will be times during the day when your anterior cingulate cortex fails, leaving you vulnerable to the pull of those cues. Maybe you're eating because it's Friday night, or because your favorite show is on, or because you're on vacation, or because you're reading. These are not just habits for you—the things that, in the past, you have associated with eating can become like gravitational forces, keeping you trapped and circling in their orbit.

Emotions are also very powerful cues. Whether due to boredom, anger, celebratory joy, fear, insecurity, grief, loneliness, frustration, happiness, or sadness, emotional eating is as common today as mindless eating. We even call it "comfort food," for goodness' sake! And these messages start young.

A few years ago, I took my then-two-year-old on a car trip to visit Niagara Falls with a friend of mine who is also a Bright Lifer. We had a great adventure, but when it was time to get back in the car and head home, my daughter refused to get clicked into her car seat. She started arching her back, pushing against the car seat, and wailing—typical behavior for that age. My poor friend watched the mayhem for a few minutes, then started rummaging in our cooler. She handed me a plastic baggie full of crackers and raisins to give to her.

I tossed it on the floor of the car and finished clicking in my daughter. Then, as I climbed into the front seat to drive off, I took a deep breath and decided to offer a different type of food—food for thought. As lovingly as I could, I said to my friend, "Do you see what you just did? Maya wasn't *hungry*. She was *angry* about having to get clicked into a car seat. You wanted me to give her food. But that had nothing to do with what she was upset about. Do that often enough and you'll teach your kid that negative emotions are a cue to eat."

She was blown away and, as we drove back, we talked about how her mom had done that exact thing to her as a child. If those connections between uncomfortable emotions and hitting that dopamine release valve are hardwired in childhood, over time, emotions become the cues that predict food rewards. When a child is crying a parent never says, "Would you like some broccoli?" It's usually a cookie, a cracker, or another sugar- or flour-based treat that's offered.

People talk a lot about emotional eating. According to this way of looking at it, if emotions are your cues, then they're your cues. All of us sign trackers have a range of cues that pull us toward food, and emotions are usually in the mix there somewhere. People frequently say to me when they start my Boot Camp, "I just need to heal this emotion; then I won't overeat anymore." I would posit that you might simply need a system that teaches you how to break the behavior of acting on the cue.

One last thought about this. If you're a goal tracker and food is rewarding but the cues that predict it aren't, then it will be pretty easy for you to stop overeating. You have to give up the excess food, and that's that. But if you're a sign tracker and you get powerfully pulled in by the myriad cues in life that predict food rewards, then quitting addictive eating is an entirely different ball game. Your whole life has become one big series of cues to eat, the pull is invisible and incredibly strong, and escaping can seem nearly impossible. Impossible, that is, until you adopt a method of eating that was designed to solve this exact problem.

Nature vs. Nurture

Before we end this discussion of sign tracking and goal tracking, I want to address one lingering question you might have been pondering: Is addictive susceptibility genetic, or environmental? Scientists have done the research and it turns out that, in rats at least, it's powerfully genetic. Sign-tracking rats mated to other purebred sign-tracking rats nearly always give birth to baby sign-tracking rats. Goal-tracking rats mated with purebred goal trackers nearly always give birth to baby goal-tracking rats.[6] Addiction runs in their genes.

Then researchers did another ingenious experiment. They took two nonaddictable, goal-tracking rats and mated them together, so they got a whole litter of nonaddictable babies. Then they took some of the babies away and raised them in isolation, which is stressful for a rat and mimics emotional trauma to a human child. Many of those babies turned into addictable rats.[7] Other researchers showed that stressing the rats by making food rewards uncertain could also result in goal-tracking rats acting like sign trackers.[8]

Essentially, put under enough stress, a genetically nonaddictable rat can be turned into an addictable rat. It doesn't happen every time, but it happens often enough.

I don't know about you, but I teared up the first time I read that. It answered a lot of my own questions about why some of us are more prone to addictions than others, why some of us end up on the end of the bell curve, where we don't want to be. It also started to address a lot of questions on the forefront of addiction research, like why so many combat veterans develop addiction after serving tours of duty.

Nature and nurture are interesting topics, but at some point, spending too much time wondering why you became susceptible and when your food problem originated amounts to navel-gazing if you're not also embarking on a proven program of action to solve the problem. And the biggest obstacle to succeeding in that program of action, funny enough, is probably not going to be the big food manufacturers or your mother-in-law's freshly baked cookies.

It's going to be you.

But not all of you, just a part of you. A part I like to call the Saboteur. Outwitting your Saboteur has everything to do with understanding how your impulses originate in the brain. And that's what we're going to cover next.

Case Study: Corina Flora

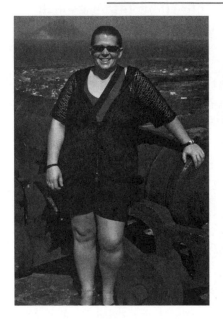 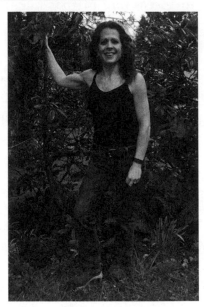

Highest Weight: 225 pounds
Current Weight: 134 pounds
Height: 5'4½"

I have struggled with my weight for as long as I can remember. I was nine years old when I went on my first diet. I can't even tell you how many times I've tried to lose weight in my lifetime. I've tried Weight Watchers more than once; Atkins; Overeaters Anonymous; The Zone Diet; Dr. Oz's diet plan; Dr. Phil's diet plan; Suzanne Somers's diet plan; the Blood Type Diet; and the honey, lemon, and cayenne fast. I know there have been others, but I can't remember all of them. I lost the most amount of weight when I turned vegan; that lasted 10 months, but I just couldn't sustain it. I got down to 163 pounds, but then I gained it all back, plus more!

I'm definitely a food addict, a 9 on the Susceptibility Scale. I used to eat when I was happy, sad, stressed, bored . . . you name it. I could always find a reason to eat. After having two kids and juggling the demands of a very busy life—their school and activities, running my own business, working on my degree in podology, and maintaining a household—my weight crept up to its all-time heaviest of 225 pounds.

I looked happy on the outside, but on the inside I was so disappointed that I couldn't get my act together—not only for me, but for my family. Emotionally and physically, I was tired a lot of the time. Once I was finished with work and the many things that had to be done every day were done, I would often relax in front of the TV for hours and snack.

Then my mom sent me the links to Susan's *Food Freedom* video series. When I watched them, they totally made sense to me. All of the programs I had tried before had usually focused on food or exercise, but none of them had really focused on the behavioral part of eating. That was the missing link for me.

I worked through the program exactly how Susan teaches it. I did not break my Bright Lines once throughout my whole weight-loss journey. After just the first few weeks, I started feeling great. I loved not having to worry about my food—there was nothing to obsess about. I lost 11 pounds in my first week and had so much energy I started organizing and cleaning my house! I was finally starting to feel in control of my life again.

My journey hasn't been without struggles, of course. At first, going out to restaurants was a bit stressful. The fear of the unknown was difficult. Would they be able to accommodate me? Would I get enough food? But the celebrations and rewards I've experienced with Bright Line Eating far outweigh the struggles.

When I started, my goal was to lose the weight before I turned 40 and to finally put my food issues behind me. I was tired of feeling like I was missing out on things in every aspect of my life, especially with my husband and kids. Well, I'm happy to say it happened. I reached my goal weight the day before my fortieth birthday! I was so thrilled.

I've experienced many physical benefits as well. I have a lot more energy. I don't have the same kind of aches and pains as I did before. Getting up off the ground and simply moving is effortless now. When I go out for walks, I want to push myself more because it feels so good. I easily wake up at 6 A.M. every day—I don't have to drag myself out of bed.

I have a new sense of self-confidence and take pride in how I look. I love that my body finally reflects how I feel on the inside: accomplished. Food was one aspect of my life I could rarely control and, when I did, it didn't last long. Now I have the confidence to take chances I might not have taken before. I feel like more business opportunities will open up for me. I'm excited to see what will happen.

My thinking about food has totally changed. It doesn't feel like I'm on a diet or like I'm following a particular program anymore. It's not that I *can't* eat certain foods—truly, I don't *want* to. I'm never white-knuckling around food because I never give my taste buds a reason to want it. The enjoyment that I might get for a few moments is not worth the sugar crash and the addictive behavior that will follow. Nothing tastes as good as living Happy, Thin, and Free feels!

CHAPTER FIVE

THE SABOTEUR

For four chapters, we've been talking about how eating the Standard American Diet can hijack and rewire the brain. But what does this sound like in your head as you're going around, living your life? Many of us who've tried to lose weight in the past can relate to feeling like we have two parts to our personalities, each with different agendas. There's the part that wants to get thin and stay that way and is bound and determined to manage our behavior to be successful this time . . . finally. Then there's another part that whispers in our heads, *It's just a little taste . . . you deserve to have some . . . it won't count . . . go ahead, no one's watching . . . you'll start again tomorrow.* In Bright Line Eating, we call that voice the Saboteur. It's the part of us that tries to derail our best plans and intentions.

Where does it come from? Why does it try to undermine us like that?

In this chapter, we're going to find out.

What Is Consciousness?

Many years ago, while I was at the University of Rochester completing my Ph.D., I had the pleasure of talking with one of the most preeminent neuroscientists of our time, Dr. Michael Gazzaniga, after a talk he gave at the medical school. He was telling me about one of the most interesting things to have emerged from decades of neuroscience research on the brain: the understanding that consciousness doesn't arise from one place, biologically speaking. Rather, each part of the brain that governs an area of function also gives rise to the consciousness about how that function feels. This means the motor cortex doesn't just make you raise your hand, it also produces the awareness of how it *feels* to raise your hand. The olfactory cortex doesn't just help you smell, it gives you the awareness of what it feels like to do it.

In essence, many parts of the brain "talk" to us. What's important to understand is that, even in a very healthy person with no psychological issues, each part of the brain advocates for its own interests and agenda. We often perceive this as "thinking." When we get a blister, we get a signal to our brain from our foot, which manifests as a voice inside our head that says, "Ouch, this really hurts. I need to stop walking." We weigh that request coming from our heel, but frequently that just isn't an option. So we tell our heel, "I know it hurts, but I can't stop right now, so hang in there."

But if we're not savvy about how consciousness is distributed in the brain, when the conversation happens between parts of the brain, we can misperceive the origin of these thoughts. We can perceive all those messages as coming from one integrated "I." "I'm on a diet." "I want to have a drink at the party." "I'm not supposed to drink on the diet." "I don't want anyone looking at me funny if I don't have a drink." "Fine, I'll have the drink." But really those messages telling you to have the drink you know will derail your weight-loss efforts are no more from "yourself" than your heel telling you it hurts.

What I want to teach you to do in this section is learn to recognize the voice of the Saboteur and be able to talk back to it the way we talk back to our bodies all the time, such as when we push through walking with a blister, teaching with a headache, or being stuck in traffic when we have to pee. Regulating your eating is no different once you understand how the brain works.

An Experiment

We discussed the brain stem a little in Chapter Two, when we looked at where leptin, the hormone that signals "I'm full and it's time to get moving" was blocked. To recap, the brain stem is the most primitive part of the brain. It controls our basest functions, like dilating or constricting our pupils, making urine, and taking in oxygen. Those with sleep apnea probably know that the brain stem is what wakes you up enough to take a breath. It's where our primal drive to survive originates.

The brain stem, too, has a voice.

And I want you to meet that voice.

So I want you to do a little experiment. Right now, please. What I want you to do is to decide that you're going to hold your breath for two minutes. Decide it. For real. Decide that everything you ever wanted to have happen in your life is right on the other side of that successful two minutes. Relax, get prepared, set a timer and . . . go.

Now, as you hold your breath, what I want you to notice is the narrative in your mind. At some point within the first minute it's going to turn from "I got this" to "this is crazy" and maybe even "screw this."

Then you "decided" to breathe, right? You judged that nothing bad was really going to happen if you took a breath, and you were uncomfortable, so a voice in your head said "Just do it. Breathe."

The point is, *you* didn't. Decide, that is. Your brain stem did. *But it got what it wanted by convincing you in your own voice.*

Consciousness is not a unitary phenomenon in the brain. Different parts of the brain create their own consciousness, but to us they all sound like "me." This is where inner conflict comes from. Even incredibly primitive parts of our brain talk to us in our mind with our own voice when they need to direct our behavior. They reason with us, and they win. We think we've chosen our behavior and decided to take a certain action, but that's an illusion. It felt like you decided to take a breath, but you did it because your brain demanded oxygen. *You* didn't actually have much say.

The Left Hemisphere Interpreter

What I want to look at now is what happens in the brain *after* you've taken that breath you vowed you wouldn't take.

In 1967 Dr. Roger Sperry and the aforementioned Michael Gazzaniga—then a Ph.D. student under Sperry at Caltech in Pasadena—published a groundbreaking study, "The Split Brain in Man," in *Scientific American*.[1] The subjects of their study were four men who had been the recipients of a surgery meant to cure severe epilepsy. The surgery involved severing a band of fibers called the corpus callosum that connects and carries signals between the right and left hemispheres of the brain.

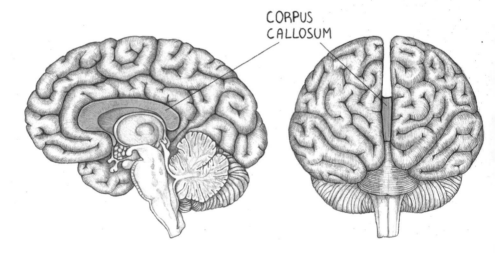

CORPUS
CALLOSUM

Ten men had undergone the experimental surgery when Sperry and Gazzaniga did their research, but only four men participated in the study. After the surgery, their epilepsy improved vastly. But they now had brains whose two halves couldn't talk to each other. Sperry and Gazzaniga wanted to understand exactly what the repercussions would be.

What they already knew was that the left hemisphere is the seat of speech and analytical capacity, and that the right hemisphere helps recognize visual patterns. They also knew that the brain and the body crisscross—the left hemisphere controls the right side of the body, and the right hemisphere controls the left side of the body. It's called "contralateral control." Even the eyes work this way. So, once the corpus callosum is severed, if you show an image only to the right visual field, only the left hemisphere sees it. And vice versa. Fascinating, right? It gets better.

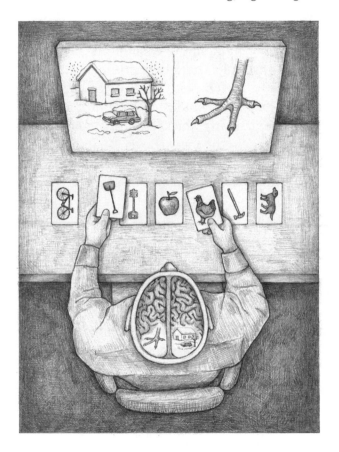

The man in the picture sees a chicken foot in the right visual field, and is processing it in his left hemisphere. Simultaneously, he is seeing a snow-covered house scene in the left visual field and processing it in his right hemisphere. The task he was supposed to accomplish was simply to pick the card on the table that related to what he saw.

What happens next is that, because the right hemisphere sees a snow scene, it tells the left hand to pick up the picture of the snow shovel. Simultaneously, the left hemisphere sees a chicken foot and tells the right hand to pick up the picture of the chicken. But then, when the man looks back and forth at both of the cards in his hands, both hemispheres get to separately see them and process what he just did.

Then the scientists ask him to explain his choice.

Language is seated in the left hemisphere, the part of his brain that has seen the chicken foot, so what the man *should* have said, and what the scientists *expected* him to say is, "I saw a chicken claw, so naturally I picked out the chicken, but I have no idea why I picked up the snow shovel. That makes no sense."

But that's not at all what he said. Instead he said, "The chicken claw goes with the chicken. And you need a shovel to clean out the chicken shed."[2]

And the researcher says, "Really? *That's* why you picked up the shovel?" And the left brain says, "Yes."

Then the researcher asks, "Do you remember having that thought when you picked up that card?"

And the left brain replies, "I do. Yes, I remember having that thought."

Of course that's nonsense. His left hemisphere had no such thought. The part of his brain responding to the researcher's question wasn't even the hemisphere that selected the card. But the truly baffling thing is that *he never realizes that he's lying to himself.* In trial after trial, each of the four men spun confabulations to explain their choices without once picking up on the fact that they were doing it. They never even noticed that they were behaving strangely. They completely believed the stories they were telling.

It turns out that the job of the left hemisphere is to make sense of our choices, and it's going to come up with an explanation—no matter how bizarre our behavior or how far it has to stretch the truth. For this reason, it's come to be known as the Left Hemisphere Interpreter.[3] And it works exactly the same, even in people whose corpus collosum hasn't been severed.

The implications of this couldn't be more profound.

Let's take a moment to connect the dots.

As we covered in Chapters Two and Three, our brain stem and our nucleus accumbens generate powerful, driving motivations. If leptin is blocked, the brain stem sends the message "Eat!" If the dopamine receptors in the nucleus accumbens have down-regulated, they demand "More!"

In our own voice.

And then the Left Hemisphere Interpreter comes along and rationalizes our behavior.

So as we go about our lives, making four or five failed attempts to lose weight each year, making choices that are 100 percent incongruent with our goals, with our vows, and with the future we most want for ourselves, the left hemisphere is busy contriving stories to explain those choices regardless of whether they make sense. We ate the cupcake because we've had a long day, we're at a birthday party, we deserve a treat, and why start the diet now anyway when we have a cruise coming up in a month that we'll want to enjoy?

Those are stories the Left Hemisphere Interpreter fabricates to explain the behaviors that originate as demands coming from other parts of the brain. Demands we have no power to deny when we don't know where they're coming from.

No wonder we can't lose weight.

The Saboteur and Self-Perception Theory

It goes deeper. One of the most corrosive side effects of the way modern "foods" and patterns of eating have hijacked our brains is the impact of all this on our self-perception—how we judge ourselves at the deepest level.

Dr. Daryl Bem of Cornell University first posited self-perception theory in 1972.[4] It was a radical theory at the time. It said that we come to know who we are by watching our own behavior. Previously, the scientific community thought that self-knowledge drove our behavior. Most people still assume that we know who we are inherently, and that we then pick behaviors in alignment with that sense of who we are—in alignment with our beliefs, values, attitudes, and political leanings.

Dr. Bem disagreed. His research showed that we form opinions about ourselves exactly as we form opinions about others—by judging our behaviors. No difference. If a friend is always late, you eventually decide they are not only an unpunctual person, but probably also a disrespectful one. You do the same to yourself.

The psychology of this is very, very upsetting for someone who is high on the Susceptibility Scale and who has fallen prey to year after year of resolving to eat differently only to have the brain stem and nucleus accumbens hijack their resolve. They have eaten foods that they promised themselves they weren't going to eat, or had second and third helpings when they said they were only going to have one. Over and over again.

This is the scary thing: If we set goals to eat just *these* foods and not *those* foods, and then we watch ourselves "decide" otherwise in the moment, we watch ourselves lie to ourselves, rationalize our behavior, and betray our highest intentions. Over time, we come to decide that we don't like ourselves, we don't value ourselves, and, in some cases, that we loathe ourselves. It is faulty wiring in the brain that demands that we eat, then talks us into thinking that we chose to, and ultimately makes us conclude that we have deep-seated psychological problems because we can't keep our word.

Some psychologists propose that "it's not what you're eating, it's what eating you." I say it's the opposite. You'll never get to your goal weight by trying to love yourself more or by working on self-acceptance. That's not where the fundamental issue lies.

Think of it another way. Do you know yourself to be kind to others? Accomplished at many things? Able to take care of yourself well in many areas? All of that is what's real. You love yourself just fine. The problem isn't what's eating you. It's what you're eating.

Case Study: Tami Oren

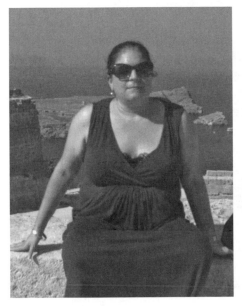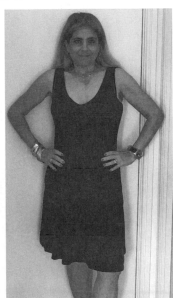

Highest Weight: 202 pounds
Current Weight: 123 pounds
Height: 5'3"

When I was two years old, my parents divorced. In Israel in 1976, that was not common. They both formed new relationships right away and I went to live with my mom and my stepdad. My parents did not have the same view of my upbringing and both families led very different lifestyles. It caused a lot of tension and disagreements over the years and fundamentally infuenced me. When I was eight, I was sent to live with my dad and his new family, and the day I moved to live with them, heartbroken over being made to choose between my parents, I started eating addictively. Even at that young age I didn't like being overweight, but the more I felt bad about myself, the more I ate and the bigger I got.

I loved food. I absolutely loved food. It was probably my primary relationship. I was raised in Israel, and at that time we didn't really have fast food, and we didn't have snacks in the home like most people have today. And we didn't have sodas. But I was always obsessed with quantities. I loved big portions. I remember always worrying that there wouldn't be enough for me. I'd eat a lot and then finish whatever no one else wanted. Food was so important to me that I'd save my allowance to go eat out. My mother was very controlling, so I would take what little money I had and buy foods that weren't allowed, like big slabs of chocolate or candied nuts. Food was so much more than nourishment to me. In fact, it was everything *but* nourishment.

My first actual diet started when I was 12. I saved my pocket money and purchased the book *Diet for Girls*, which was mostly about calorie restriction. Very 1986. But at 14 my family moved to a kibbutz, which was another trauma. We had to eat at communal tables, and I remember panicking, thinking *"There's not going to be enough food for me!"* I started eating whatever I could again. I wasn't massive as a teenager, but I was always ashamed of my body and wanted to change it.

Then, from age 18 to 20, I did my Israeli military service. I lost all my excess weight at the beginning and kept it off for the whole two years. But when I got back to the kibbutz, I put on 22 pounds in two months and the weight just kept coming. I was big, unhappy, and ashamed. I went on my first proper diet when I was 23, just before my wedding. I lost 27 pounds but after my wedding I regained it all—plus some.

From there my life followed a typical cycle of trying restrictive diets and losing the weight only to regain it, plus extra. I tried one diet that prescribed quite serious calorie restriction during the day, but then in the evening allowed you to eat anything up to 800 calories. Even with the nightly binge I felt deprived, and I hated it. I tried another diet that started with 100 days of food-replacement shakes only, coupled with neurolinguistic programming and cognitive behavioral therapy to address food addiction. I lost 66 pounds, but when I started introducing foods again it was impossible for me to control my portions and I put it all back on.

Then I got pregnant. After my son was born I just hated my body so much. My stomach felt like a bottomless pit, like I would never know fullness—ever. So I thought the best thing would be bariatric surgery. I went to see a surgeon for my fortieth birthday and he looked at me and said, "I've never seen a fat vegan before. If you can be vegan, you can do anything. You're just not being strong-willed enough." I was so humiliated I binged for two months. And then a friend posted Susan's *Food Freedom* videos on social media. She saved my life. For years I had thought, "What's wrong with me?" I watched the videos and thought, "I can solve this. There *is* a solution." Then I joined Bright Line Eating and discovered there was nothing wrong with me, only with what I'd been eating.

It wasn't easy to begin with—I was really miserable because of the quantities. For five weeks I felt like I was starving. I was really tired and fatigued, but I stuck with it because I knew I was drowning and this was my rescue boat. After seven weeks it became bearable; then, after three months, it became easy. Now I can't imagine my life any other way.

Everything has changed: I don't hate myself and I don't hate my body. I've never experienced those feelings before in my life, ever. The madness isn't there anymore. I've found peace.

And I've really met myself now. The best version of me has emerged from this process.

Part II

THE BRIGHT LINE EATING SOLUTION: BRIDGING THE WILLPOWER GAP

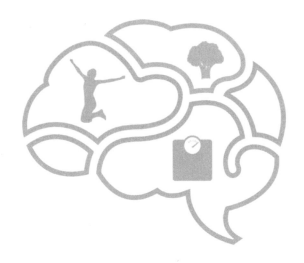

A quick note: If you have just bought this book and flipped to this chapter because you want to "cut to the chase," I strongly encourage you to go back and read the first five chapters. You will find out *what* to do in this chapter to get Happy, Thin, and Free, but if you don't know *why* you're doing it, your chances of success are much lower. That's just a scientific fact.

CHAPTER SIX

THE FOUR
BRIGHT LINES

Now you understand how your brain is blocking you from getting Happy, Thin, and Free and why every diet you have committed to so strongly in the past has ultimately failed you. Insulin levels have crept up, blocking leptin at the brain stem so the all-important signal "Ugh, no more eating. I'm full!" simply doesn't arrive. And if your dopamine receptors have downregulated, too, then it's taking more and more sugar and flour throughout the day to deliver the same feeling of "okayness." In the past you've pledged and committed to eat right, but fighting against your brain takes every drop of focus and effort you've got. Sometimes, despite all of your resolve and best intentions, the strains of the day wear away at you and the Willpower Gap is right there, waiting. Add to all that a voice in your head that is constantly manipulating you, urging you to make an exception "just this once," and a consciousness that has watched you struggle and concluded you're not trustworthy, so why bother . . . It's no wonder you have felt hopeless about the prospect of ever losing all your excess weight and keeping it off. In truth, up until now, it *has* been hopeless.

The Way Out

There is only one long-term, sustainable solution to this mess that I have ever seen work. It worked for me, and I have seen it work for thousands of others. Give up sugar and flour. Completely. Get them out of your system quickly and definitively.

It's possible you want to throw this book across the room.

It's also possible you were given this book by someone who has lost and kept off a hundred pounds or more, so you're willing to keep an open mind.

Either way, you're probably asking me right now, "Isn't that *extreme?*"

To which I reply, "I'll tell you what's extreme." Each year in the United States alone, over 70,000 people have to get a limb amputated because of their Type 2 diabetes.[1] *Seventy thousand people.* Their doctors have warned them it's coming, but it doesn't matter. They can't stop. They eat until they lose a limb. *That* is extreme. *That* is how powerful this addiction is. Giving up processed drug-foods isn't extreme. What's extreme is the way our society eats—and the consequences we've decided we're willing to tolerate as a result.

And *of course* the answer is to quit. When someone is losing critical lung function because they smoke two packs of cigarettes a day, we don't tell them to moderate their smoking. We tell them to quit.

"But how?" you're asking. "Cigarettes are easy to avoid. Food is everywhere! And I have to eat to survive and there are special things I love to eat that have sugar and flour in them and I don't know if I could give them up forever and you've just pointed out how hard it is to stick with anything . . ."

I hear you. And it's okay to feel panicked—that's actually coming from the dopamine receptors in your nucleus accumbens. They are about to get their supply cut off and they don't like it. Not one little bit.

Which is why I'm happy to tell you that this program is stronger than they are. Your brain *will* heal, and there's a very,

very bright future ahead of you. Relax. It won't be nearly as bad as you think.

Bright Lines to the Rescue!

After I'd been in a right-sized body for over a decade and had spent years and years helping people in my community lose hundreds of pounds as a spiritual service, I discovered Roy Baumeister's book *Willpower*.[2] He's the scientist who performed the famous radish experiment described in Chapter One. Toward the end of the book, on page 185, he talks about Eric Clapton's alcoholism and says this:

> He needs the help of "bright lines," a term [borrowed] from lawyers. These are clear, simple, unambiguous rules. You can't help but notice when you cross a bright line. If you promise yourself to drink or smoke "moderately," that's not a bright line. It's a fuzzy boundary with no obvious point at which you go from moderation to excess. Because the transition is so gradual and your mind is so adept at overlooking your own peccadilloes, you may fail to notice when you've gone too far. So you can't be sure you're always going to follow the rule to drink moderately. In contrast, zero tolerance is a bright line: total abstinence with no exceptions anytime.

I was on fire. *Yes!* I thought. I had been living by Bright Lines for years in relation to drugs and alcohol, but had never heard this term before. I loved it. The mental image it conjured up almost had a spiritual feeling to me, like those sharp beams of sunlight that break through clouds and make my heart fill with bliss.

But then Baumeister goes on to say, "It's not practical for all self-control problems—a dieter cannot stop eating all food."

I was stunned. I thought, "Oh, Roy, *fumble!* Can't you *see?* Bright Lines are *perfect* for food!" I stared at that paragraph for what felt like ages. I was trying to assimilate the fact that *Roy Baumeister*, one of the most preeminent psychologists in the world, with over 30 books and 600 publications to his name, believes that you can't use Bright Lines for food because you have to eat to live. Yes, you have to eat to live. But you don't have to eat *doughnuts* to live. It was then that I truly grasped the chasm that existed between everything I knew to be true about the science and practice of effective weight loss and the state of thinking in the rest of the field. I let it all sink in. Not many days after I read that paragraph, the words *Bright Line Eating* came to me during my morning meditation session, and I resolved to write this book.

So. Bright Lines. Clear, simple, unambiguous boundaries that you just don't cross. We've arrived, finally, at the heart of the matter.

The most important contribution of the Bright Lines is that they bridge the Willpower Gap. Bright Lines give you clear rules for what you can—and can't—put in your mouth. And the result is that your eating choices become automatic. You don't have to think about them. There's no decision to make. It doesn't matter that it's 4 P.M. and that you have a tray of doughnuts in front of you. You will stand there knowing *exactly* what you are going to eat next, and those doughnuts won't be it. Bright Lines enable you to stop thinking about food, and to stop grappling with those 221 food-related choices a day we mentioned earlier. There is only one choice: respect the Bright Lines.

Bright Line Eating, as I've devised it, consists of four Bright Lines: Sugar, Flour, Meals, and Quantities. In this chapter, I'm going to outline each Bright Line in depth and explain the science behind why they work.

1: SUGAR

This is really the cardinal Bright Line. Without it, none of the others are effective, because you have to take sugar out of the equation to allow the brain—and therefore the body—to heal. To be clear, by sugar I mean all ADDED sugar. It appears as dozens and dozens of names on ingredient lists, including but not limited to: cane sugar, beet sugar, date sugar, brown sugar, powdered sugar, evaporated cane juice, rice syrup, corn syrup, high-fructose corn syrup, honey, agave, maple syrup, molasses, sucrose, dextrose (indeed, anything ending in -ose), maltitol, glycerine, malted barley extract, and maltodextrin. Any food containing any of these ingredients has to be eliminated because all refined forms of fructose and glucose hit our insulin system harder than our bodies were designed to withstand. Elevated baseline insulin levels then block leptin, leading to insatiable hunger and sedentary behavior. And the sugar pounds our dopamine receptors, leading to downregulation and overpowering cravings. In order for your brain to heal, your insulin and dopamine systems must be allowed to rest so they can recalibrate back to their original settings.

Artificial Sweeteners

Artificial sweeteners are a scourge. True, they have zero calories so the body cannot use them for fuel, but they impact the insulin system just the same as sugar. The sweet taste hits the tongue and causes a dopamine surge and insulin response even though no corresponding calories are forthcoming.[3] And, in 2014, researchers discovered an additional mechanism by which artificial sweeteners cause glucose intolerance: by altering our gut microbiota.[4] Finally, research shows that, in some organisms, artificial sweeteners mimic a starvation state in the brain, leading to a 50 percent increase in food consumption.[5] Don't be fooled. Artificial sweeteners will absolutely derail your weight-loss success. By artificial sweeteners I mean saccharine, NutraSweet, aspartame, sucralose, xylitol, sorbitol, and, yes, stevia and Truvia. In addition, many nonfood products containing artificial sweeteners, like diet soda and sugarless gum, will keep you hooked on the behavior of putting something in your mouth as a crutch to get through the day. Take a deep breath and let them go.

Fruit

The good news is that fresh fruit is just fine. In fact, fruit is wonderful! I am happy to say that you can eat any and all varieties of whole, fresh fruit. The fructose in fresh fruit doesn't impact the brain and body like refined sugar does because when you eat a piece of fruit, you eat fiber as well. Fruit's "fiber lattice" is composed of soluble and insoluble fiber that slow the absorption of the fruit's natural sugar into the bloodstream, blunting insulin and dopamine responses.

What we shouldn't eat is dried fruit, fruit juice, or blended fruit. In each of these, the sugar content is more concentrated than the fiber lattice can inhibit. Imagine sitting down and eating six fresh apricots, for example. It would probably take you quite a few minutes and you'd most likely start to get bored with eating them before you could even get through them all. Now imagine eating six dried apricots. You could do that in seconds, and the only thing you'd be thinking is, *"MORE!"* Remember, we want to keep that part of your brain, those dopamine receptors, quiet.

I get asked all the time whether juicing and smoothies are allowed. The answer is no. Here's why. The soluble and insoluble fiber in fruits and vegetables work together to form a barrier that keeps the fructose from rushing through your gut lining and flooding into your bloodstream. The fiber barrier is kind of like the roof of a thatched hut. The *insoluble* fiber is not digestible—think of it as the twigs or bamboo that you'd use to make the roof of the hut. The *soluble* fiber does gradually dissolve, like the packing mud on a hut. Once you take that whole fruit—or vegetable, as the case may be—and put it in a blender or juicer, you shred the fiber lattice, leaving all that fructose and glucose free to hit your system as fast as if you'd consumed a piece of candy.

Cravings

The next thing that I'm usually asked is, "If I quit sugar, won't I have cravings?" Yes, you will. At the beginning, Bright Line Eating is very similar to quitting smoking. But the cravings will go away. Not instantly, but by the end of my eight-week Boot Camp, 84 percent of people report having few or no cravings anymore—ever. Some people, like me for instance, experience cravings for a while longer, but I promise, *I promise*, they go away. The craving is just the last-ditch effort of your hijacked brain to get you back on the sauce. But you will become stronger than that. The next few chapters will help you put systems in place to get through those cravings so your brain can keep healing and you can reach your goal weight. And, finally, stay there.

2: FLOUR

The second Bright Line is flour. In my opinion it's the wiliest. Bear with me on this, because it's vitally important. Most people are so wary of sugar that they let flour sneak in under the radar and sabotage their success. In the twenty years I spent working with and observing people in various 12-Step food programs, I saw this happen over and over again. People gave up sugar, but they kept eating flour. Or they gave up white flour but kept eating brown flour. So they stayed heavy. Or they gave up wheat flour, but they ate oat flour. So they stayed heavy. Before I developed Bright Line Eating, I tried giving up sugar without giving up flour. What happened is that I mourned the loss of my cookie dough, because there's no cookie dough without sugar. But then it dawned on me that I also loved *pie crust dough.* So I started to eat that. I also started focusing on pasta, quesadillas, corn chips, chow mein, pizza, pot stickers, English muffins, and more pasta. I ate a lot of French fries and potato chips, too, which technically don't have flour in them—but I know now that the inside of a white potato is the molecular equivalent of straight flour, just pure glucose without fiber. Essentially, my brain cued me to escalate my flour intake to compensate for the dopamine loss from sugar, so I actually gained weight. It's a classic mistake. I urge you not to make it.

We don't have research on this yet, but I believe there are individual differences in whether the brain prefers to get its fix from sugar or flour. In my experience, about 80 percent of people are primarily sugar-focused. But there's a slice of the population, the other 20 percent, who will openly admit that they don't like sweets much at all—just don't take away their bread. Those percentages are just my guesstimate from having worked with so many people. I'd love to see a study done on it.

The science of flour addiction is in its infancy. We know that flour raises insulin levels,[6] but we don't have the smoking gun of flour flooding the dopamine receptors. YET. But let me remind you of that anecdote about putting sauce and cheese on broccoli. No one has ever driven out in the rain at 3 A.M. to get that. Why do people rate pizza as the *number one* most addictive food in existence?[7] It's the flour.

All Flour

Just as with sugar, the Bright Line for flour is ALL flour. It's not about the type of plant. It's not about gluten. It's about *surface area*. When the grain is processed, ground down to make flour, the surface area of each particle gets multiplied exponentially. This is true for "whole-grain" flour, too. When the surface area is increased, our digestive enzymes have a field day accessing the glucose and it hits the system too fast and too hard.

My friend, Dr. Alan Christianson, gave me a great analogy for this. He said he thinks about the digestive process as akin to melting ice. Eating a whole-grain food, like brown rice, for example, is like taking a huge square block of ice and leaving it on a driveway to melt. It will, but slowly, over the course of many hours. Eating brown rice flour, in contrast, is like sprinkling ice shavings all over a hot black driveway. They melt on contact.

Sugar and flour affect the body in slightly different ways, which is why it's important to give them up in tandem. Sugar primarily breaks down into glucose and fructose. Flour breaks down into just glucose. Fructose can only be processed by the liver, which is why we're seeing such high incidence of fatty liver disease in our culture. Flour hits *all* the cells. Think about that. A full-body assault.

3: MEALS

Eliminating sugar and flour is a good start, but if that's all you do, odds are you won't be successful long-term. Eventually you'll fall prey to the Willpower Gap and your efforts won't last. This is where the Bright Line for meals comes in. When regular meals become part of the scaffolding of your life, it takes the burden off willpower. A lot. When you set up a schedule of eating three meals a day at regular mealtimes—breakfast at breakfast time, lunch at lunchtime, and dinner at dinnertime—not only does eating the right things become automatic, but passing up the wrong things in between also becomes automatic.

At first you may find breaking your long-standing habit of eating between meals to be quite hard, because you're probably not used to prioritizing eating at mealtimes. And you're probably not eating *enough food* at mealtimes. But the Bright Line of meals is a habit that can be established fairly rapidly, and from then on it will serve you well. It may even improve the lives of those around you. As I said earlier, as a culture, we have lost the concept of real meals. We graze all day. There is no time of day now when food is not on offer. And, if you or your loved ones are prone to food addiction, like those sign-tracking rats, this means that your whole day has become one long series of magnetic cues that pull you in and result in food going into your mouth without you necessarily even being aware of it. In short, if you allow yourself to eat between meals, you're sunk. You'll never get thin that way. Or happy or free, for that matter.

The Bright Line for meals means eating three beautiful, abundant, delicious meals a day—with absolutely nothing in between. (Bright Line beverages are fine; see page 149 for a list.) If you're thinking, "But I get hungry at four o'clock! I need a snack!" I can honestly tell you, after working with thousands of people, you don't. Or, rather, you *won't*—once you get your blood glucose stabilized and your insulin under control. Three meals a day will be fine. Even people who start Bright Line Eating with a diagnosis of hypoglycemia typically find that it resolves quite quickly, that it was caused not by an underlying physiological disorder, but rather by the sugar and flour they were eating.

There are situations where more or fewer meals per day are called for, but in these cases the Bright Line for meals—no grazing and no snacking—still holds, it's just that the number of meals varies. Here are some examples. When I was pregnant with twins, I ate six meals per day. But they were *meals* that I planned out and ate with attention. (And, three years later, when I was pregnant with just one baby, I happily and healthily ate just three meals a day throughout the entire pregnancy.) And the day I climbed Half Dome, I ate six meals. But just on that one day—during shorter training hikes leading up to the big climb, I stuck to my three-meal schedule. Sometimes, but not always, gastric bypass patients have to eat smaller, more frequent meals. It depends on how much time has passed since the surgery and how their body responds to the Bright Line Eating food plan. Bodybuilders and athletes on a serious training regimen are another group that may need more than three meals. In addition, some of my clients with eating disorders who come to Bright Line Eating to get their weight *up* can't actually handle the portion size of Bright Line meals and have to break them up at first. As I said, there are noteworthy exceptions, but, in my experience, the vast majority of people are served well by three meals a day.

Eating meals on a regular schedule also confers a long list of powerful health benefits. It dramatically increases the fasting window—the number of hours that you go without ingesting any food—up to roughly 11–14 hours (a 13-hour fasting window is accomplished if you finish dinner by 6 P.M. and eat breakfast at 7 A.M. the next morning), and this increases fat loss,[8] improves energy levels, and facilitates a good night's sleep.[9] A nice long fasting window also increases something called autophagy,[10] which is the process by which your cells recycle and repair their broken and poorly working parts, boosting your protection against infection and disease.[11] And eating meals at *consistent times* improves insulin sensitivity, lowers cholesterol, and supports fat loss.[12]

When it comes to diet and exercise programs, the cultural zeitgeist leans heavily toward recommending snacking, so it might be wise for us to take a moment to debunk some popular myths about eating throughout the day. The first myth is that eating small meals throughout the day keeps your metabolism revving and increases energy expenditure. There's a lot of research on this, and it's simply not true. Your metabolic rate will be the same whether you eat three bigger meals or six smaller meals per day. It might even be *better* with fewer, bigger meals.[13]

So what are the supposed benefits of snacking? After all, I cannot think of a single diet or eating plan (other than Bright Line Eating and a handful of 12-Step food programs) that advocates three meals a day with nothing in between. *Every* other eating plan, that I'm aware of, builds in snacks. Maybe the thought is that snacks keep you from getting hungry and are just *necessary*, that without them people would want food all the time and feel deprived. Well, there's research on this, too, and actually, in some populations at least, it's the reverse. It's eating all day long that keeps people thinking about food, obsessed with eating, and feeling hungry again right after putting food in their mouths. Eating at regular meal times alleviates all that.

So in practice, what does the Bright Line for meals look like? Well, here's a picture for you. In the morning, shortly after waking, you will sit down for a Bright Line breakfast. Eating while seated is important. There, on your table, you set out the food you've planned to eat. It does not happen in your car, on the sidelines of soccer games, at the movies, or on your couch.

It is time to eat when you're at the table. By shifting the cues your body uses to recognize acceptable times for consuming food, you shift them *away* from everything else that used to trigger you.

Lunch may have to be at your desk, but this can work if you eat at a set time every day. Again, I ask you to be mindful. Turn off your computer. Maybe give thanks. The same for dinner. Consider weaning yourself off of the habit of eating dinner in front of the TV. Entertainment can be a cue to relax, or to share a laugh or cry with friends and family, but it shouldn't be a cue to eat.

Resetting the brain this way isn't easy at first in our on-the-go culture, but it's worth the effort. Again, primarily because once your brain is really clear about where it eats, it becomes really clear about where it doesn't, and those endless cues for us sign trackers fade into the background.

4: QUANTITIES

The fourth and final Bright Line has to do with Quantities. This is the Bright Line that clicks everything into place and ensures that your weight will melt off and leave you in a right-sized body. Postmenopausal? On medications that increase your hunger? Obesity run in your family? Hypothyroidism? No worries, the Bright Line for quantities has got your back.

The quantities of Bright Line meals are generous, but they are finite. Remember that the majority of adults no longer receive reliable signals to stop eating from their brains and are no longer able to compensate for the extra calories they've consumed. And almost no one who is overweight these days is able to consistently choose portions that will result in them losing all their excess weight and keeping it off. So we take your judgment out of the equation.

I recommend a digital food scale. Yup, I suggest you weigh your food. Sound crazy to you? I know how you feel. I used to feel the same way. Initially, when weighing and measuring was first suggested to me, I balked. It sounded obsessive and extreme. For *years*, I refused to do it. And I kept struggling with my weight. But then I tried it, and what I found was that weighing my food with a digital scale gave me *tremendous* psychological freedom. I didn't have to think about what I ate after I ate it, or wonder if I had had too much or too little. I knew I was getting the right amount of food. The value of that is that now, when I hear a voice in my head telling me to eat more, I *know* it's the Saboteur.

I weigh and measure my food precisely because that kind of precision can be automated. Every morning when I weigh my 1.0 ounce of oats, I weigh out exactly 1.0 ounces. Not .9 and not 1.1. Because when you think, "Oh, that's close enough," you activate a part of the brain that is vulnerable to the Saboteur. Is today's "close-enough" the same as yesterday's? "I had .1 oz. less oats than usual this morning—so I can have a little more fruit with lunch." No. None of that. We're committing to automatic and consistent.

BLTs

In my world, BLT doesn't stand for a type of sandwich, it stands for "bites, licks, and tastes." And they're the enemies of Bright Lines. I don't taste sauces bubbling on the stove; I'm not popping a piece of red pepper in my mouth as I'm making a salad. I commit not to taste my food until I get to the table. In the early days, when I couldn't actually be in the kitchen without licking spatulas and nibbling on crusty bits at the edge of the frying pan, I even put Scotch tape over my mouth to break the habit of eating unconsciously. Avoiding BLTs is important because you want to have real integrity with your food, and also because it's shocking how easy it is to nibble your way up a pant size.

The History of "Bright Lines" and Food Addiction

The principles that I evolved into Bright Line Eating were first introduced to me at a 12-Step meeting for food addiction. I started adding 12-Step food meetings to my schedule of other 12-Step meetings at the age of 21, just one year after getting clean and sober. And what I want to share is that, while I think the support and healing process of 12-Step programs can be invaluable, I was not handed the blueprint for getting Happy, Thin, and Free at meeting one. It took me *eight years* of attending meetings on a near-daily basis to experience lasting success. There are as many different philosophies about how to manage compulsive overeating and food addiction in 12-Step programs as there are 12-Step food programs themselves.*

For the first several years, I attended a program that was focused on support; its philosophy was not to prescribe a specific food plan. People would come to meetings and share their short-lived triumphs or what they had binged on. They found comfort and mutual understanding, but most people stayed heavy.

Eventually I moved on to another group that did have strict guidelines, and those guidelines helped me lose all my excess weight, for which I am profoundly grateful. However, that program was very rigid, and, as I shared in the Introduction, it nearly broke up my marriage. In fact, my husband left me for nine months over it. Clearly, the way I was being guided to work that program was out of balance with my life. But I still *needed* both structure and community.

I was confronting a common paradox of the 12-Step food community: If a program is relaxed enough to accommodate a busy life, acknowledging that people have kids and other priorities, the less likely it is to work for any given attendee. The programs that seem to work really well for long-term weight loss tend to be rigid, even fanatical, in their approaches. That said, for people who are willing to submit entirely to their structure, *they do work.*

---

* Which is to say, at least seven. To my knowledge, the major 12-Step food programs include Food Addicts in Recovery Anonymous, www.FoodAddicts.org; Food Addicts Anonymous, www.FoodAddictsAnonymous.org; Overeaters Anonymous, www.OA.org; GreySheeters Anonymous, www.GreySheet.org; CEA-HOW, www.ceahow.org; Anorexics and Bulimics Anonymous, www.aba12steps.org; and Recovery From Food Addiction, www.RecoveryFromFoodAddiction.org.

But the really interesting thing that I noticed, over the years, was something going on outside the 12-Step rooms, in the general population. Only a tiny percentage of the people I knew who needed and wanted to lose weight were interested in exploring a 12-Step solution to their problem. For a long time I assumed that they would come around—or would keep eating their way through a miserable existence if they didn't come out of their "denial." But gradually, I started to think differently. I realized that, first of all, food addiction is a continuum, as described by the Susceptibility Scale, and many of those people simply didn't have problems extreme enough to make them be willing to attend several weekly meetings and stand up in front of a room full of people and say they were food addicts. But also, 12-Step programs simply aren't for everyone. Some people take issue with the God-based approach to recovery, and others just aren't joiners. This finally sunk in for me one sunny day in Rochester, New York, when I was walking with a dear friend who happened to be obese. She explained to me all the reasons why 12-Step programs were not her thing. She'd never go. I get that now. I also watched her weight yo-yo for well over a decade, and I very much wanted her to have a road map that would help her be successful.

Bright Line Eating exists because it seemed like there needed to be an alternative. One that had enough structure to be permanently effective, but that could be flexible enough to allow people with busy lives to participate successfully. One with a strong commitment to science, and that would explain the reasons behind the guidelines, not just seem to assert them arbitrarily.

At the same time, yes, it is possible for some people to get Happy, Thin, and Free by going to a 12-Step program. There are many of them, and I can't make a blanket statement about what works best, because a) it depends on your particular needs, preferences, and situation, b) odds are that not every program will have meetings near you, and c) the meetings for one program can be very different in different cities. But I can tell you what to look for if you decide to check out a meeting. If there are a bunch of slender people there who show you pictures from when they were heavy, have a sparkle in their eye, and are eager to help you find a sponsor, you've found a home. If you go and there are lots of people in the room who are still quite heavy and have been attending meetings for years, move on.

So what, exactly, are the differences between Bright Line Eating and a 12-Step program? Bright Line Eating is based on science, features a powerful Online Support Community, and conducts cutting-edge research to help shape our global understanding of the obesity pandemic. If you're a 10 on the Susceptibility Scale, you might find a home in a 12-Step program that feels really comfy. You might want and need a sponsor, and prefer the face-to-face support of that live community. And meetings are free if finances are your driving concern. Also, you don't need to choose. Plenty of people have benefited from participating in both.

I am a huge fan of *support* and *resources*. Whatever works for you to get and stay Happy, Thin, and Free is what you should do.

Case Study: Scott Steinhorst

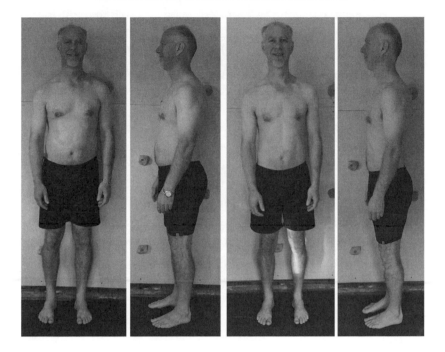

Highest Weight: 184 pounds
Current Weight: 145 pounds
Height: 5'9½"

I was fit and trim through college, but I had an irritable stomach. I eventually discovered the symptoms were greatly improved by eating refined carbs and always keeping food in my stomach. This led to the habit of eating too much, too often.

For ten years after college, I worked a desk job as a mechanical engineer and software developer. Over that time, I slowly gained weight until I reached my highest weight of 184. I repeatedly tried to start exercise programs and learn more about eating healthy. My diet did improve over time, but I had little success with weight loss or regular exercise. I didn't feel like myself, and was very unhappy with my weight.

In 2001 I lost 30 pounds on the Body-for-LIFE program, but I didn't continue with the diet after the program, and the exercise plan fell away before long. A year and half later I quit my desk job to stay home with my kids and gradually my weight started to yo-yo, going up five or ten pounds in the fall and winter, then dropping every spring when I did a three-week cleanse. But I became more and more aware of how little choice I sometimes felt I had over what or how much I ate.

The winter of 2014–2015, I gained more than usual. Spring and summer passed with my energy and mood lower than usual. I completely failed to improve my diet, complete that three-week cleanse, or otherwise lose the weight as I had before. I knew I needed to make a change, I just couldn't manage to do it.

In the fall, I joined the Bright Line Eating Boot Camp. Now I have the success with my food choices, my weight, and my health that I had been trying so long to achieve.

At first, making a food plan and writing it in my food journal each night was hard. Figuring out how foods matched up with the food plan and figuring out what to eat was also hard. But I made a deep, inner commitment to stay perfectly within the Bright Lines. Perhaps this resonated so strongly with me because of Susan's emphasis on personal integrity and the negative psychological effects of failing with food.

By halfway through the Boot Camp, organizing food and keeping my food journal was much easier—I understood the food plan and became acquainted with a variety of meals and foods I could eat. I found the simple preparation and arrangement of whole foods in Bright Line Eating much easier and much less time-consuming than anything I had tried before, and I easily integrated it with feeding my family.

My long-term brain fog cleared up very early on and has never returned. I felt weak, but not tired. In fact, I easily switched to decaf coffee, whereas I'd previously used caffeine and eating to keep up my energy throughout the day. A few weeks into the Boot Camp my blood sugar stabilized and I started experiencing the new—and odd—feeling of having steady energy all day long.

I love to weigh my food. I take such great comfort from knowing I am, every meal and every day, eating exactly the right amount of healthy food. Without my scale I would live back in the land of crazy, always wondering, *Should I have more? Is this too much? Am I losing weight? Gaining weight?* Occasionally I will scoop too much cooked oatmeal into my breakfast bowl and it will occur to me to leave it there and then my mind starts to wind up . . . *Should I? Shouldn't I? Will it matter? Will it lead to more?* Instantly, it becomes obvious how quiet my mind usually is and how messing with the formula is a quick trip to crazy land. No way do I want anything to do with that! It doesn't affect my weight as much as it affects my mind. Out comes the bit of extra oatmeal, and I go back to the land of quiet freedom.

So thin, clearly. Free, certainly. But happy? I've long fallen in and out of episodes of depression—in recent years I've become more and more affected by the seasonal affective disorder (SAD) symptoms here in Seattle. This winter, since I began Bright Line Eating? Nothing. Not a whiff of the depression thing, or of the SAD fall/winter thing. And for that I am very, very grateful.

Sometimes I feel a little pull now and then from non-BLE foods, especially from foods other experts recommend as "healthy," like smoothies, juice drinks, kombucha, or recipes packed with super nutrients. I quickly remind myself they're express tickets to that life I don't want to live anymore.

Food used to take up so much room in my life that I felt a sense of failure, like I was living someone else's life in someone else's body. Now I feel a sense of integrity. I feel successful. I feel like I'm living life as the best version of myself.

CHAPTER SEVEN

AUTOMATICITY: YOUR NEW BEST FRIEND

When people are first introduced to the concept of Bright Line Eating, their initial questions—once they've gotten over the shock of being asked to give up sugar and flour—usually include: "But doesn't sticking to those Bright Lines require willpower?" "How on earth am I going to do that?" "Isn't this just another diet telling me which foods *not* to eat?" I tell them that this is absolutely not just another diet. The reason people lose their excess weight and, much more important, *keep it off* with this plan is that Bright Line Eating is carefully constructed to shift eating behaviors out of the part of the brain where decisions are made, the prefrontal cortex, and into the part of the brain where things are automatic, the basal ganglia. Bright Line Eating is a complete and integrated system. It takes some willpower to set up, but requires little to no willpower at all after that.

Consistent repetition of Bright Line Behaviors makes them become automatic. This is vital, because we are trying to keep your Saboteur quiet. We don't want you ever making *decisions* about what to do next. We want to set you up so that the crucial components of every Bright Line day are automatic. This accomplishes three goals: it keeps you at goal weight, takes the burden off willpower, and quiets the food chatter in your mind. There's nothing for your brain to figure out, puzzle through, or make a decision about. Choosing the right foods just becomes a habit.

Habit in the Brain

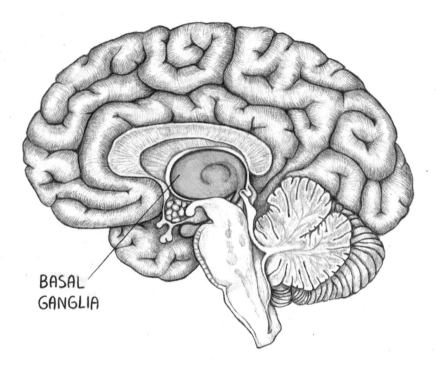

BASAL
GANGLIA

The brain evolved to make certain behaviors automatic; this frees up other parts of the brain for making decisions. Think of it this way: kneeling in the dirt to tend crops or to make a fire left us vulnerable to predators. If we could perform those actions without consciously thinking about them, we could remain on alert for rustles in the underbrush and have enough mental bandwidth left to quickly decide whether it was a jackal or another tribe member approaching. The basal ganglia is the part of the brain responsible for that automaticity.

What This Looks Like

The difference between using willpower and using your automatic brain to accomplish something is tremendous. If you've ever tried adding a new habit to your morning routine—exercise, five minutes of meditation, reading a page out of an inspirational book—you've probably experienced what it's like to forget, get too busy, or decide to skip it "one time." But now think about brushing your teeth. I don't know about you, but I predict in a year's time I will have accomplished brushing my teeth in the morning 365 times regardless of traveling, illnesses, or work commitments. It's nonnegotiable. What's more, I don't have to think about it. I spend exactly zero energy worrying that I won't get it done. Contrast that to how my young daughters, Alexis, Zoe, and Maya, feel about the same task. They need daily reminders and cajoling to get it done. Why? It's not automatic for them yet.

Do you remember when you first learned to drive a car? And your first attempt at merging with the flow of traffic on a highway? Do you remember the heart palpitations? The *focus* it required? And now you can probably do it while drinking a latte and simultaneously changing the radio station. The point here is that once something becomes automatic, it frees up *tremendous* cognitive resources for other things. And you don't have to think about the behavior *at all* to get it done.

The best part, in terms of staying true to your regimen, is that it will eventually feel uncomfortable when you *don't* do it. One of my friends got an oral night guard very late in life and for two months she hated it. Now she can't fall sleep without it. There's no doubt about it—investing a few short months in muscling through the habits of Bright Line Eating until they become automatic is tantamount to giving yourself a gift that will arrive on your doorstep every day for the rest of your life—a lifetime of living Happy, Thin, and Free.

How Long Will It Take?

This brings us to the question of how long it takes to form a new habit. How long will it take for you to go from consciously remembering to weigh your food, sit to eat at a table, approach your usual Dunkin' Donuts location and just keep on driving, to doing these things as a matter of course, without even giving them a second thought? Let's use me as an example. I'd say I have a very full life. I don't *think* about Bright Line Eating any more than I think about brushing my teeth. I just *do* it. But I did have to make an investment to get here.

The fact is that getting Happy, Thin, and Free required me to focus really hard for a while on getting my food right. I wish there were a world in which people like me—and maybe you— could eat whatever we wanted whenever we wanted all the time and live Happy, Thin, and Free. That world may have existed 1,000 years ago, but, alas, it's not the world we live in now. So, if you want what's on offer here, you're going to have to invest some energy for a while to get your food right, too.

How long does it take for us to form a new habit? Researchers wanted to know, so they asked subjects to start a new eating, drinking, or activity behavior and record whether they carried out the behavior each day, and whether it felt automatic to do it. On average, it took 66 days for the new behavior to become 95 percent automatic.[1] Note that this is in contrast to what you might have read or heard about in the media. No, it does not take a mere 21 days to form a habit. Nor even 30. The true number is 66 days. However, that's just an average—the range is immense. On the low end, automaticity was achieved in as few as 18 days, and on the high end, 254 days.

That means you're going to have to give yourself between 18 and 254 days to focus on this pretty intensely. Keep in mind, though, that the people in that study were asked to add *one* new behavior to their life. Getting Happy, Thin, and Free is going to require adding several new behaviors, breaking many long-standing habits, and, for some, kicking an addiction, too. That's a big ask.

Bunny Slippers

So, during this period before Bright Line Eating becomes automatic, I want you to be very aware of the stress you will be placing on your willpower, and do everything you can not to overtax it. Reduce obligations at work if possible. Be conscious of the things you do that tap your resources, like moving your kids through their bedtime routine, and plan your Bright Line Meals accordingly. Either eat beforehand or have it laid out ready and waiting for you afterward. If you always got through a dreaded Wednesday staff meeting by relying on the pastry tray, eat your Bright Line lunch beforehand. And make sure you are getting enough sleep each night. Sleep is a powerful willpower replenisher.[2]

Overall, in the early days, the rule of thumb is to travel gently. Imagine yourself going through your day wearing bunny slippers. That's the attitude I want you to take toward this early weight-loss phase. You may feel very tired for a few months. That's normal, and it will pass. Drink a lot of water and know that the fatigue is real, but it's temporary. The time for feeling fantastic and being out in the world is coming—later. At the beginning, give yourself permission to be gentle with yourself. And a key part of that is . . .

No Exercise

Yes, you read that correctly. Bright Line Eating is a no-exercise plan. During the initial habit-formation phase, I strongly discourage people from increasing exercise levels. Doing so depletes willpower, which is dangerous to your long-term goals. It will be the straw that breaks the camel's back.

Once you are living Happy, Thin, and Free, and Bright Line Eating is an ingrained habit, adding exercise can have wonderful mental and physical benefits. Studies have shown regular exercise improves memory, attention, and learning capacity.[3] It staves off Alzheimer's and other dementias.[4] It boosts the immune system.[5] It strengthens your muscles and your bones, can help with balance, and protects against osteoporosis.[6] It strengthens your heart. It increases self-esteem.[7] It even improves your sex life.[8] And once you're in a nice, slender body, it helps you to maintain that physique. Practically the only thing it doesn't do, it turns out, is help you lose weight.

It's true. Exercise won't make you thin. In one study, Dr. Timothy Church at Louisiana State University[9] assigned 464 overweight, postmenopausal women into four groups. Each was assigned to work out an average of 0, 72, 136, or 194 minutes per week at an intensity of 50 percent of their peak VO_2. There were no dietary modifications. At the end of six months, the exercisers hadn't lost any more weight than the zero-minute control group. As the amount of exercise increased, the body's "compensation" increased—essentially, the exercisers got hungrier and their will-power was more depleted. This means their Saboteurs were that much more successful in talking them into a post-workout latte and muffin.

When you look closely at the science of exercise, the weight-loss benefits just aren't there. And yes, I am aware that people lose a lot of weight on *The Biggest Loser*. But they don't keep it off,[10] and that's the point. The reason to *not* exercise during the weight-loss phase of Bright Line Eating is that it's already going to take every last drop of focus and willpower you've got to establish thick, consistent, and totally habitual Bright Lines. If you're distracted or depleted in any way, you'll cut corners, let exceptions weasel their way in, and the whole endeavor will unravel. But if you give yourself the gift of this short period of time to really concentrate on this, you'll reap the benefits for the rest of your life. In my view, weight loss should be a one-and-done thing—a very brief and unique time of your life. Let's get that weight off you once, now, and fast. Then you can go back to exercising and enjoy it in your right-sized body for the rest of your life.

If you're still worried, I promise you that thousands of people in my Boot Camps have lost their excess weight without exercising. I have seen it with my own eyes. And I've seen the opposite, too.

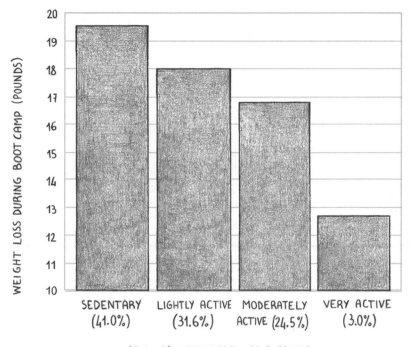

Average weight loss

SELF-DESCRIBED LEVEL OF EXERCISE

Participants in the study that generated this chart were asked to characterize their level of exercise during the eight-week online Boot Camp. As it shows, increasing levels of exercise were associated with *decreased* weight loss during the period when people were learning new eating habits and trying to make them automatic. Other groups have found this, too. In a study at the Pennington Biomedical Research Center, researchers showed that during the first eight weeks of their study, the diet-only group lost about 5 percent of their initial weight while the diet-plus-exercise group lost only 3.5 percent.[11]

It's also important to recognize that exercise is part of the pathology for many of us. And here it gets tricky, because exercising is also a very healthy, empowering thing to do. And a thing we *should* do. But in my experience, many of the regular exercisers—not all, but many—who land in the Bright Line Eating Boot Camp are pretty wacked-out about exercise. Overexercising to compensate for overeating can be an addictive cycle in itself. And they don't even realize they're doing it. But try to take it away from them, even for a few short months, even for a very good reason, and the neuroses start to surface.

What we want at Bright Line Eating is to get to a place where exercise is valued for all its health benefits, but also totally and completely uncoupled from weight loss in our minds. They truly are not related.

There are exceptions to the no-exercise rule: If you've been doing it every morning for 15 years and you do it as reliably as you brush your teeth, you get a free pass for obvious reasons. If it's not taxing willpower, it won't interfere. Similarly, if you've been diagnosed with depression or anxiety, the benefits of exercise may just outweigh the cost. A depressed or anxious brain may prevent you from breaking free. As a side note—we'll get into this more in Chapter Fifteen—you may find that your depression and/or anxiety disappear with Bright Line Eating. That's not a promise; it's a prediction based on my own experience and that of many others.

Automaticity

Bright Line Eating is structured on the prevailing science about what is "automatizable." Some things are readily automatizable, and others are not. Learning to eat three meals a day is an easily automatizable behavior. Learning to eat six is much, *much* harder. Yes, when I was pregnant with twins I ate six meals a day. But it was hard. I'd had many years of Bright Line Eating under my belt by that point, and I returned to three meals a day as quickly as I could, because I wanted that automaticity back. Six meals felt like a juggling act.

When we deviate from our food plan and the actions and strategies I'm going to share with you in Part III, we leave ourselves vulnerable to the Willpower Gap and the Saboteur. It's that simple. I'm going to teach you in Part IV how and when it's okay to deviate, with things like moving our fruit from lunch to dinner because we're going to a wedding and we want to choose fruit instead of cake. That's a sensible, strategic plan. But there's a huge difference between altering your food plan once, or even permanently, in a structured way—during a pregnancy, say—and just casually swapping foods and categories daily based on the prevailing winds of your whims. That is a setup for failure. For many people, eyeballing portions works the same way. It invites the Saboteur to try to convince them they haven't had enough. Believe me, I know. Sometimes I travel without my food scale— and at those meals you'd better believe my Saboteur will ask me if maybe I need more food. Weighing imprecisely is another area for caution. You simply don't want the assessing, deciding part of your brain to have to get involved at all.

An Invitation

Over the coming months, you'll have tons of automatic behaviors to break and tons of other automatic behaviors to develop. It is going to sap nearly all your available willpower to do this and to do it well. So what this means is that you're going to have to carve out space. Slow down. Be gentle with yourself. Recognize that this period of weight loss is going to be a unique, intense, and, in many ways, truly precious time. You're giving yourself an incredibly valuable gift.

If you set up Bright Line Eating right, you will end up with automaticity, and that will pay dividends for the rest of your life. It will result in nearly every dream you've ever had for yourself coming true. But if you don't carve out the time to do it right, if you insist on exercising too much, working too hard, or otherwise set yourself up to cut corners, the system won't get implemented properly, you'll hardwire in exceptions here and there, and this will go down in your weight-loss history as one more attempt that didn't stick.

I invite you to decide right now to commit to the program as it's laid out—no wiggle room, no exceptions. You have to *trust*. It's time to be unstoppable. It's time to give yourself this gift.

Case Study: Jan Deutsch

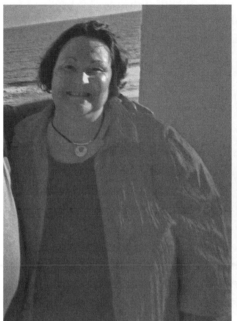 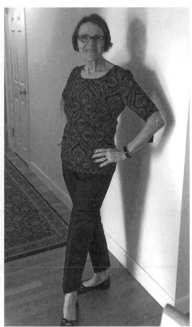

Highest Weight: 333 pounds
Current Weight: 141 pounds
Height: 5'6½"

I had a body that was fully mature by age 14, which made me feel very self-conscious about myself. I weighed 135 pounds and was almost 5'7", by no means overweight, but, to my mind, I was fat. So I started Weight Watchers. By the time I was 17 years old, I was in great shape . . . but then off I went to college and gained about 20 pounds during freshman year. After that, I spent years on a roller coaster of losing 20 pounds, gaining 20 pounds. Then came my three pregnancies, which initiated an even steeper roller coaster of repeatedly gaining and losing 40 pounds.

At one point, I did successfully lose 80 pounds on a supplement diet. But the very day I achieved my goal, I began eating junk food again. I think that was my lowest, saddest point. I felt like the ultimate failure. I just gave up, and wouldn't even think of dieting for the next eight years. During that time, I gained back all the weight I'd lost and MORE, for a total weight gain of 153 pounds. I ate whenever I possibly could. Whether I was happy or sad, it didn't matter—I ate for comfort.

By no small miracle, I met my bariatric physician when I was at my highest weight—333 pounds—and that's when I accepted that I'm not a weak-willed, lazy person. I was addicted to sugar and flour. What a relief!

I initially lost a large amount of weight by following a reduced-calorie diet—no sugar, no high-fructose corn syrup, and no white flour. But one day, I was looking for something sweet to eat and opened a container of raisins. Over the weekend, I ate the whole container—and started to experience that out-of-control feeling again. Luckily, a few days later, I heard Susan Peirce Thompson being interviewed by Katie Mae. Her words resonated so deeply that I immediately abandoned all flour, reduced my artificial sweetener intake, only ate three meals a day, and started weighing and measuring my food.

I think the two aspects of Bright Line Eating that had the biggest impact on my success were eating only three meals each day and committing to my food the night before. I had always been a grazer, eating almost every hour, on the hour. I never ate until I was full at meals because I wanted to save room for at least one or two snacks in the evening. The hardest part of the plan for me was eliminating snacking, as that meant my nighttime routine of several mini-meals would no longer be an option. It took about three or four weeks to get used to that. I drank lots of tea, kept my hands busy, and stayed out of the kitchen.

I should mention that I was eating the Whole-Food Plant-Based way, where the philosophy is as long as you eat WFPB foods, there is no need to restrict quantities. But not for me! My compulsive overeater brain would tempt me to eat more and more. This is why the Susceptibility Scale made so much sense to me. I'm a 10 on the scale—I don't know when to stop. Even after reaching goal weight,

I continue to weigh and measure my food because it gives me freedom. I know that what I have on my plate is exactly what I need. No second-guessing.

Today, I wear a size six or eight—in anything from jeans to dresses—and I actually weigh ten pounds less than when I got married. My life has changed dramatically over the past six years. At my worst, my triglycerides were through the roof; my HbA1c rose to 6.9 (in the diabetic range); and my knees, hips, and back ached from the extra stress and strain I was putting on them by carrying 193 extra pounds. Today my blood work is exceptional and my body doesn't ache. In the past, I was either shut out of—or shut *myself* out of—so many activities that required physical effort. Now I have participated in several 5K runs and a 10-mile walk. I kayak and canoe, and I can ride a bike, too. One of the most memorable moments for me in the last year was fulfilling a wish I first made about 20 years ago, in Vermont. I was out on a golf course and saw glider planes swooping overhead. I thought, *"Oh, I'd love to do that someday."* But then I looked down at my 300-pound body and said to myself, *"No way."* There was a weight limit for glider passengers. Well, in August 2015, I fulfilled that dream. It was so exhilarating to soar over the mountains. Dreams really do come true.

Part III

THE ROAD MAP: GETTING STARTED

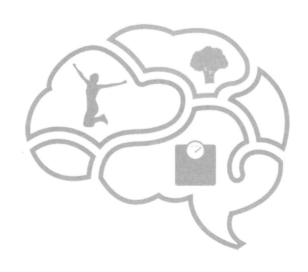

CHAPTER EIGHT

THE WEIGHT-LOSS FOOD PLAN

I imagine you're eager to read up on what you're going to eat. Don't worry, there are lots of choices. Ok, I hear you asking, "But will I *enjoy* them?"

Yes.

Eventually, you will. Maybe even immediately. The foods you can eat on this plan are tremendously varied because Bright Line Eating is a complete lifestyle. It's not about living on lettuce for six weeks—or grapefruit. It's about eating real food that is good for your brain, in quantities that produce—and then sustain—your weight loss.

There are three pieces of good news on the food-enjoyment front. First, if downregulation was an issue for you, as your dopamine receptors heal, you are going to find that you're able to taste your food in a way you may not have been able to for years. Second, every cell in your taste buds dies and is replaced by a brand-new taste bud cell *every two weeks*,[1] so as you detox, your taste buds will be going through their own evolution, and in very short order your food will taste AMAZING. I say this to you as someone who used to eat a whole lot of cookie dough and who now eats a whole lot of vegetables. I love my vegetables—they taste incredible and leave me full and satisfied. But, no, my appreciation for them did not happen overnight.

Third, what you'll find is that your food will taste better because you'll be coming to each meal with an eager stomach and a body that truly wants and needs fuel.[2] It turns out that has a huge impact on the way the food tastes. I don't know about you, but in the past, I was always topping up my tank before the fuel light ever came on. And, because my body didn't really need the fuel, I had to seek out hyperpalatable taste-bombs to placate my worn-out taste buds. No more. When you're truly physiologically hungry, abundant, colorful, healthy food tastes phenomenal. It feels like your body is saying, *"YUM! Thank you!"*

One warning: as you read through the food plan for the very first time, you may find yourself having a strong reaction to what seems like a complex, rigid, overwhelming system. That is very common. I promise it will get easy and start to feel simple very, very quickly. Food is just complicated because there are so many great options. Reading about it all can feel like trying to get a drink of water from a fire hydrant. I suggest you read this section through and then take some deep breaths, calm yourself down, and tell yourself to just try it for a while and see. No commitments, just an experiment. Thousands of people have done this successfully, and there's no difference between them and you. This plan works beautifully if you follow it.

There's another thing I need to prepare you for up front, and it might surprise you to hear me say this: This food plan is *not* designed for optimal nutrition. It's designed to be a wide, lenient plan that will succeed at getting you Happy, Thin, and Free. My intention is that, after you have your transformation, or somewhere along the journey, you will be inspired to select more and more choices that are more and more healthy . . . that you will naturally get curious about nutrients, and will want to swap out iceberg lettuce for arugula or kale. But since I'm asking you to give up sugar entirely, give up flour entirely, never snack, and weigh and measure your quantities, I'm not inclined to force more limitations immediately if they're not actually necessary for the initial weight loss. There are other experts whose sole objective is to help you get maximally healthy through optimal nutrition—we don't need more experts doing that. It's being done well already. I see my job differently. I'm here to get you into a right-sized body and to give you back full authorship of your own destiny when it comes to the food you put into your mouth. At that point, making even healthier food choices will be something you can do if you want. And, of course, if you want to aim for maximal nutrition starting from day one, that's great, too. All the most nutritious foods are on the plan, so there will be no barrier to your success.

As you read over the Weight-Loss Food Plan, you may wonder how it can be that this one plan works for everyone. That's a question I get a lot. The answer is that the differences in people's sizes and metabolisms simply manifest in how *fast* they lose their excess weight, but once they get down to goal weight they will indeed end up on different maintenance plans based on their metabolic needs. Note, though, that the Weight-Loss Food Plan doesn't recommend the same amount of food for everyone every day. For starters, at all three meals, men get more protein than women. But also, you yourself can vary the amount of food you're eating quite simply. For example, you can choose nonfat cottage cheese for your protein or cashews for your protein, but you'll take in nearly *four times* as many calories with the cashews. Hence, we talk about making "light" or "heavy" choices within the food plan, based on your needs or whether you know you're going to be taking a long hike that day.

Another point: if you are currently attached to a philosophy of eating, like paleo, Nutritarian, vegan, or gluten-free, I promise that you can easily adapt this food plan to your needs and continue to adhere to the guidelines of that program. Since 2012, I have been a predominantly plant-based eater and Bright Line Eating has kept me beautifully slender—for all the years that I included meat and dairy in my diet, and all the years since. As long as the philosophy isn't based on eating cookies every night, there's a way Bright Line Eating can make it work.

And finally, as you start to read this, I invite you to surrender and simply keep an open mind. The most successful people in Bright Line Eating are those who just decide to trust the plan and do it as outlined. After all, nothing you've ever tried before has gotten you where you've wanted to be, right? Thousands of cases show that this road map works. Trust.

The Weight-Loss Food Plan

If you have at least ten pounds to lose, this is where you'll start. You'll stay on this plan until you get down to goal weight. If you are at goal weight already, or have fewer than ten pounds to lose, read through this chapter and then read the beginning of Chapter Fourteen, about the Maintenance Food Plan, for instructions on how to get started.

The Weight-Loss Food Plan		
Breakfast:	1 protein	
	1 breakfast grain	
	1 fruit	
Lunch:	1 protein	
	6 oz. vegetables	
	1 fruit	
	1 fat	
Dinner:	1 protein	
	6 oz. vegetables	
	8 oz. salad	
	1 fat	

How long it will take you to get to goal weight, of course, depends on how much weight you have to lose and how quickly you lose it. There is a wide range for how quickly people lose their excess weight doing Bright Line Eating, but on average people lose 1–3 pounds per week, meaning some lose less and some lose more, but most fall within that range. It's important to note here that, contrary to widespread belief, there is actually no scientific evidence showing that it's better to lose weight slowly.[3] I say get it off.

Also, I have seen again and again in Bright Line Eating that people's goal weight shifts once they have seen their bodies respond to the plan. When I was struggling with my weight, I started off aiming to get down to a size 8. Size 4 was outside my realm of comprehension. I used to think—hand to God—I was big-boned. Nope. My bones are bone-sized. I'm a size 4. So set a goal, but don't be surprised if that number shifts down for you in a few months.

Once you begin approaching goal weight, you'll want to consult Chapter Fourteen on the Maintenance Food Plan. That's where I map out for you all the details on how to transition your food plan to slow—then stop—your weight loss.

Breakfast Grains

Breakfast Grains	
Precooked Hot (weigh 4 oz. after cooking) Dry—Cold or Hot (weigh 1 oz. dry, then cook)	
Potato (4 oz. cooked)	Oatmeal (1 oz. dry)
Sweet potato (4 oz. cooked)	Oat bran (1 oz. dry)
Yam (4 oz. cooked)	Cream of rice (1 oz. dry)
Rice (4 oz. cooked)	Grits (1 oz. dry)
Quinoa (4 oz. cooked)	Cream of Wheat (1 oz. dry)
Millet (4 oz. cooked)	Quinoa flakes (1 oz. dry)

Whole grains are perfectly fine on the Bright Line Eating plan, but at first you'll only have them at breakfast. When you're close to goal weight, you'll add them to lunch, and then ultimately to dinner as well. Most standard breakfast cereals are not on the Bright Line Eating plan because they contain sugar, flour, or both. As an aside, when it comes to packaged foods, *small* amounts of sugar or flour actually are okay. Sugar and flour both have dose-dependent effects, and experience has shown that minuscule amounts won't be potent enough to trigger cravings. The rule here is that you need to read the list of ingredients in the product and if there's no sugar or flour in the *first three ingredients* then it's okay. You'll need to get into the habit of reading the ingredients list for absolutely every packaged food item you buy—but most of your food will be whole food, without a package and without an ingredients list anyway. Following this rule, there are a few commercially made cereals that will work just fine. They include Uncle Sam's original, Ezekiel cereal, Shredded Wheat, and different varieties of unsweetened puffed grains. These have no sugar or flour at all. In addition, Fiber One has been included in the Bright Line Eating food plan since the beginning. It has artificial sweetener as its 10th ingredient on the list. I'm sure there are other acceptable breakfast cereal options available in your local grocery store that are not listed here. Remember that you're watching for sweeteners of any kind—including evaporated cane juice or artificial sweeteners—or any form of flour. If you are gluten intolerant, of course you will want to find a gluten-free alternative, but be sure it does not have any form of sugar or flour listed in the first three ingredients. Quinoa flakes are my personal favorite gluten-free hot breakfast cereal.

For cold cereal, weigh out exactly 1 oz. and either eat it dry—Shredded Wheat, for example, can be eaten like crackers; this is a good option when traveling—or add milk, unsweetened soymilk, or unsweetened yogurt, which you will count as your protein. Due to their extremely low protein and calorie contents, other nondairy milks (almond, etc.) are not recommended during the weight-loss phase, although they are acceptable (see the notes on breakfast proteins below for a nice suggestion on how to split your protein if you like to use almond milk or other nondairy milks).

For hot cereal, weigh out exactly 1 oz. and then add water, typically 4–6 oz., and cook in the microwave or on the stove top until the cereal reaches the desired consistency. Alternatively, you can cook it with some kind of milk if you are using that as your breakfast protein.

Proteins

Animal-Based Proteins Typically Eaten at Breakfast (Women)	Animal-Based Proteins Typically Eaten at Lunch/Dinner (Women)	Animal-Based Proteins Typically Eaten at Breakfast (Men)	Animal-Based Proteins Typically Eaten at Lunch/Dinner (Men)
8 oz. plain yogurt	4 oz. chicken (not breaded, skin off)	8 oz. plain yogurt	6 oz. chicken (not breaded, skin off)
8 oz. milk	4 oz. turkey (skin off)	8 oz. milk	6 oz. turkey (skin off)
2 eggs	4 oz. pork (no ham cured in sugar)	3 eggs	6 oz. pork (no ham cured in sugar)
2 oz. cheese	4 oz. beef (ground beef, steak, sirloin tips, etc.)	3 oz. cheese	6 oz. beef (ground beef, steak, sirloin tips, etc.)
4 oz. cottage cheese	4 oz. lamb	6 oz. cottage cheese	6 oz. lamb
4 oz. ricotta cheese	4 oz. fish or shellfish	6 oz. ricotta cheese	6 oz. fish or shellfish

Plant-Based Proteins Typically Eaten at Breakfast (Women)	Plant-Based Proteins Typically Eaten at Lunch/Dinner (Women)	Plant-Based Proteins Typically Eaten at Breakfast (Men)	Plant-Based Proteins Typically Eaten at Lunch/Dinner (Men)
8 oz. unsweetened soy milk	4 oz. tofu	8 oz. unsweetened soy milk	6 oz. tofu
8 oz. unsweetened almond milk	4 oz. tempeh	8 oz. unsweetened almond milk	6 oz. tempeh
8 oz. unsweetened other nondairy milk (hemp, flax, rice etc.)	6 oz. beans (or 2 oz. roasted beans, like roasted chickpeas)	8 oz. unsweetened other nondairy milk (hemp, flax, rice, etc.)	6 oz. beans (or 3 oz. roasted beans, like roasted chickpeas)
4 oz. tofu	6 oz. lentils	6 oz. tofu	6 oz. lentils
4 oz. hummus	4 oz. hummus	6 oz. hummus	6 oz. hummus
2 oz. soya granules	4 oz. shelled edamame	3 oz. soya granules	6 oz. shelled edamame
2 oz. nuts (or nut butters)	4 oz. veggie burger	2 oz. nuts (or nut butters)	6 oz. veggie burger
2 oz. seeds	2 oz. soy nuts (or dry-roasted edamame)	2 oz. seeds	3 oz. soy nuts (or dry-roasted edamame)

For breakfast proteins, regular and Greek yogurt are equally suitable. The preference would be for low-fat rather than nonfat or whole-milk products, but there's no hard-and-fast rule. Nuts and seeds are only acceptable if they weren't a binge food for you; also keep in mind that they are calorically very dense, so include no more than two servings per week until you've lost all your weight. If you prefer plant-based proteins, avoid choosing almond milk, hemp milk, flax milk, or rice milk for your breakfast protein during the weight-loss phase, because the unsweetened versions are very light on both calories and protein and they won't hold you until lunch. Fortified soymilk is a better choice.

However, if you very much want to have, say, almond milk at breakfast—in your coffee or on your cereal, for example—here's a way to make that work. Split your protein serving in half, and have 4 oz. of any kind of milk, and 1 oz. of nuts or seeds (or half a serving of beans, cheese, eggs, or any other protein you like). The benefit of, in particular, the almond/soy milk and nuts/seeds combination is that one is a little "light" and one is a little "heavy," so they balance each other out perfectly. You can split your breakfast protein like this every day if you like. I do.

An important tip on lunch and dinner proteins: you always want to weigh your food *after* you cook it. For example, if you're going to eat a hamburger, don't weigh out your hamburger patty and *then* put it on the grill or in the frying pan—it will shrink down by a whopping 25–50 percent. So when you cook food, including proteins and vegetables, cook enough for several servings. You'll have leftovers, and you'll be able to weigh out your immediate serving after it's fully cooked.

Bacon is not on the food plan, primarily because it takes a ridiculously huge pile of it to get to 4–6 oz. Be very careful about processed meats like lunchmeats, hot dogs, and sausages as well. You need to read the ingredients list carefully and make sure that sugar—dextrose, etc.—flour, or some kind of starch isn't listed as one of the first three ingredients. You're much better off eating real meats—ideally organic, compassionately raised meats.

For plant-based protein, tempeh that's made out of soy and some kind of grain (like brown rice) is fine. Smoky Tempeh Strips ("fakin' bacon") are very tasty and also a good choice. Beans and lentils are some of your least expensive and most healthy options for protein and fiber, so include them often. If you eat a plant-based diet, soy nuts are great to keep in a little preweighed baggie in your purse, briefcase, or travel bag when you're on the go. You can discreetly dump them onto your salad in a restaurant to round out a meal. Dried or roasted beans, like chickpeas, are also wonderful, and can be included in the same amount as soy nuts (2 oz. for women, 3 oz. for men). I've found little snack baggies of dried chickpeas in airport gift shops and enjoyed them for breakfast with fresh fruit and some Starbucks oatmeal after a red-eye flight.

Fruit

Fruit			
Have 1 piece:	Have 2 pieces:	Have 3 pieces:	Weigh 6 ounces:
Apple	Plum	Apricot	Berries (all kinds)
Pear	Kiwi		Grapes
Orange	Persimmon		Pineapple
Grapefruit			Cherries
Banana			Mango/papaya
Peach			Melon (all kinds)
Nectarine			Fresh figs

Whenever the size of your fruit seems unusual, it's a good idea to fall back on your trusty scale and weigh out 6 oz. For example, some bananas are very small, and you may want to weigh 6 oz. of banana. Some plums and apricots are huge, so it would be better to weigh out 6 oz. rather than having two or three. For cherries, you can weigh your 6 oz. with the pits still in and not worry about the weight of the pits, or you can weigh 6.3 oz., or 6 ¼ oz. with the pits in. (Yes, I once carefully removed and then weighed the pits in 6 oz. of cherries.) Alternatively, you can use a cherry pitter and remove the pits before weighing the cherries. Note that any kind of fresh, whole fruit is acceptable, so if you're wondering about a variety that's not listed here, it's fine.

Vegetables

Vegetables—6 ounces	
Artichoke hearts	Leeks
Asparagus	Lettuce
Beet greens	Mushrooms
Beets	Onions
Bok choy	Peppers
Broccoli	Radicchio
Broccoli rabe	Radishes
Brussels sprouts	Snow peas
Cabbage	Spaghetti squash
Cauliflower	Spinach
Carrots	Sugar snap peas
Celery	Swiss chard
Collard greens	Tomatillo
Cucumber	Tomatoes
Dandelion greens	Turnip greens
Eggplant	Watercress
Green beans	Yellow (summer) squash
Jicama	Zucchini
Kale	
Starchy Vegetables—6 ounces (Acceptable but use sparingly)	
Corn	Turnip/rutabaga/swede
Parsnips	Winter squash (butternut, delicata, acorn, pumpkin)
Peas	

Note that this isn't an exhaustive list of all vegetables. Similar to fruit, there are no vegetables we don't eat in Bright Line Eating, so if it's not on this list, never fear. Have at it.

You can prepare your vegetables raw or cooked, serve them as a salad, or some combination thereof. We have a saying in Bright Line Eating: "Produce is produce." This means that if you don't feel like a salad at dinner, you can have cooked vegetables instead. When cooking, be sure to weigh your vegetables *after* you cook them, because, just like proteins, the veggies will shrink, sometimes dramatically, in the cooking process. Also be sure not to add additional fat when you're cooking. For example, collard greens should be steamed or boiled, not cooked with butter and ham hocks. If you aren't already versed in herbs and spices, they are a great way, along with onion and garlic, to flavor your food without adding fat. The exception to the "No Added Fat" rule is spray oil. You can use Pam or some similar type of spray oil (ideally the olive oil variety) to coat a frying pan or baking sheet when you sauté or roast vegetables. It's true that this will add a trace amount of fat to the food, but not significant enough to derail your weight loss. Canned or frozen vegetables are fine, but read the label to be sure nothing has been added to them. For example, canned beets are delicious, but be sure to select ones packed in water with no added sugar; similarly, find artichoke hearts packed in water, not oil. Some frozen vegetables come in a buttery sauce or have added sugar; avoid these.

Starchy vegetables are fine to count as vegetables, but be aware that their calorie count is relatively high compared to other vegetables. For this reason I recommend that you limit your starchy vegetables to two servings a week during the weight-loss phase. After you've lost your weight, you can experiment with eating them more often so long as your weight stays stable. Notice that potatoes, sweet potatoes, and yams are not on the list of starchy vegetables. They all count as grains, and you'll be eating them again at lunch and dinner when you're at goal weight. For corn, measure out 6 oz. of kernels or have two medium-sized ears of fresh corn on the cob.

Please don't make the mistake of thinking that 8 oz. of salad means 8 oz. of plain lettuce. You'd be chewing all night! You'll want to start off with a base of about 2–3 oz. of a heavy lettuce, like romaine or iceberg, or 1–2 oz. of a lighter lettuce, like spinach or spring mix. Then add salad vegetables like tomatoes, cucumbers, carrots, red onion, mushrooms, peppers, sprouts, jicama, beets, celery, etc., on top until the total weight equals exactly 8 oz. After you reach goal weight, you can add some avocado or olives as vegetables, but during the weight-loss phase it's best to avoid these, or use them and count them as your fat (see below) as they are calorically very dense. When eating out, be sure to order your salad carefully—many restaurants add croutons, cheese, craisins, fruit, bacon bits, or heavy dressing. Ask for olive oil and vinegar on the side. You can use a spoon to measure out your oil: 3 teaspoons equals 1 tablespoon. Then add vinegar to taste.

Variety is especially important when it comes to eating a lot of vegetables without getting tired of them. If you're not familiar with some of the vegetables listed here, try to incorporate a new one every week—you'll greatly expand your repertoire. Variety is not only the spice of life, it is the cornerstone of health and vitality!

Fats

Fats
Avocado (2 oz.)
Butter (1 tablespoon or 0.5 oz.)
Margarine (1 tablespoon or 0.5 oz.)
Mayonnaise (1 tablespoon or 0.5 oz.)

Nut butter (1 tablespoon or 0.5 oz.)
Nuts (0.5 oz.)
Olives (2 oz.)
Oil (1 tablespoon or 0.5 oz.)
Salad dressing (1 tablespoon or 0.5 oz.)
Seeds (0.5 oz.)
Tahini (1 tablespoon or 0.5 oz.)

You'll add one serving of fat to your food at both lunch and dinner. For lunch, perhaps you'll choose to put the fat on your vegetables. For dinner, I suspect you'll want to add oil or dressing to your salad. You can use a tablespoon measure for your fat, but I personally prefer to weigh it out on my digital food scale because it's less messy and more precise. One tablespoon should equal 0.5 oz. Be careful, though—if you're weighing oil and you pour too much, you have to be prepared to grab a paper towel and sop some up to get it back down to the correct weight. You never want to get sloppy with the scale. Don't succumb to the Saboteur who whispers in your ear and says, "It's only a tiny bit—it doesn't matter." It *does* matter. It's a matter of integrity. It's your Bright Line.

Keep in mind that there's a huge difference between healthier fats, like those in almonds and avocados, and unhealthy fats, like soybean oil or vegetable oil, especially if they're partially hydrogenated. Vegetable oil of some kind is what you'll find in most bottled salad dressings and mayonnaise.[4] If you're going to be cooking with oil, choose olive oil, avocado oil, or canola oil. If you're going to be putting oil on a salad, I suggest using flax oil. It's a wonderful source of omega-3 fatty acids, which most of us are desperately lacking in our diet. You can't heat up flax oil, though, or it will denature the molecules due to its low smoking point. If you like to add butter to your food, that's fine as long as you keep it to 1 tablespoon per meal. There are also many excellent plant-based butter substitutes. My favorite is Earth Balance

Buttery Spread. If you're going to use a bottled salad dressing, see if you can find one that uses olive oil instead of soybean or vegetable oil. The biggest red flag about bottled salad dressings is that they almost all contain some sugar or other type of sweetener, but if it's fourth or lower on the ingredients list, then it's okay. Clearly, a raspberry vinaigrette or honey-mustard dressing won't work—these will most definitely have a sweetener (maybe two) in the first three ingredients. Ranch dressings vary; some are okay and some have sugar in the first three ingredients. Most blue cheese dressings will work and many, but not all, vinaigrette dressings will work. Just make a habit of reading the ingredients list.

I also want to acknowledge that there is tremendous disagreement these days among intelligent, venerated experts on the role of fat in a healthy diet. Some experts strongly promote a diet with little to no added fat. Others say that healthy fats are a necessary and integral part of a well-rounded diet.[5] I'm aware that some people have very intense and fervent opinions about this. My views may change in the future, but as of the publication of this book, I am agnostic about the role of fat in a healthy diet. I honestly don't think there's a smoking gun in the research literature either way. In my experience, after working with literally thousands of people, the essential elements in a healthy food plan are: eliminating sugar and flour entirely, eating tons of vegetables, and having just enough fat, protein, and fiber to ground the glycemic load of each meal so insulin levels stay steady and the brain can heal. If you're doing all that, I think the body is very forgiving about the rest. Again, what I recommend is that you trust and try the plan as written. But if you have convictions about fats that make including them in your food plan untenable for you, then by all means modify it so that it aligns with your values. Similarly, if you feel you must have more healthy fat, at breakfast for instance, then substitute it in and find something to eliminate. But make your adjustment once, up front, and then keep your plan consistent from day to day. Consistency is key.

Condiments

Condiments	
Capers (2 oz. per meal)	Mustard
Cinnamon	Nutritional yeast (0.5 oz. per meal)
Herbs	Salsa (2 oz. per meal)
Hot sauce	Salt and pepper
Lemon juice	Soy sauce
Lime juice	Spices
Marinara sauce (2 oz. per meal)	Vinegar (including balsamic)

Bright Line Eating is a program of clear boundaries, not a program of asceticism or deprivation. I absolutely think food should be delicious, and that we should heartily enjoy our meals. Condiments, spices, herbs, and salt and pepper are simple and easy additions that can make a meal fabulous. Just check for sugar or flour in the first three ingredients listed on premade condiments. And do keep an eye on your use. I have known people—including myself—to go overboard on salsa, nutritional yeast, cinnamon, mustard, and balsamic vinegar, among others. When I notice myself falling into that pattern, I tend to just let that particular condiment go for a while. Generally speaking, though, condiments of all kinds are fine. Better than fine— they're wonderful! Nutritional yeast on a salad; salsa added to some simple black beans; cinnamon on oatmeal; lemon juice and soy sauce on broccoli. Yum.

A word about salt: sodium and chloride ions play important roles in cellular processes, including synaptic transmission in the brain. When you stop eating the Standard American Diet and give up packaged foods in favor of whole, real foods, your sodium intake is going to drop precipitously. If you have very high blood pressure, that's a good thing. If your blood pressure is low, though, you might feel dizzy sometimes. This can often be alleviated by drinking plenty of water and consuming a bit more salt. Contrary to popular belief, research shows that *not* getting enough salt can also have serious health consequences.[6] Unless you have high blood pressure, you may want to start salting the food you eat on the Bright Line Eating food plan. Talk with your doctor about this.

Beverages and Alcohol

What can you drink with Bright Line Eating? Let me tell you what I drink: I drink water. When I'm at a party or restaurant, I drink sparkling water with lemon or lime. The sparkling waters that have natural flavors infused in them are fine as long as they don't also have artificial sweeteners. I also drink herbal teas of all kinds. My favorites include peppermint, ginger, licorice, rooibos, and Indian-spiced chai.

Beverages that I'm *not* so thrilled about are coffee, caffeinated tea, and alcohol, but they're not equal offenders.

Coffee and Tea If you have just one cup of coffee in the morning and you choose to have some soy, rice, almond, or cow milk in it as part of your protein serving, that's fine. But if you're having coffee or tea at a nonmeal time, then it needs to be black. The issue that I have with caffeine and Bright Line Eating is that it floods the brain with dopamine. It's an addictive substance. We're trying to replenish your dopamine receptors and heal your brain here, so doing anything that's going to flood the brain with dopamine is not a good idea. It's going to keep your cravings alive. So if you're someone who drinks a lot of coffee or tea, I would say a good firm boundary is two cups a day, maximum. At some point, try to get down to one cup a day. And ideally, I would recommend you try to wean off it completely.

Alcohol Molecularly speaking, alcohol is sugar plus ethanol. Ethanol is what makes you intoxicated. When you're intoxicated, you have a low resistance for doing dumb things and making choices that you wouldn't otherwise make. Anytime you drink alcohol, you're going to be more likely to eat something that's off your food plan. So alcohol is off-limits for Bright Line Eaters because a) it's sugar, and will keep your brain from healing, b) it reduces your inhibitions, and c) it strengthens your Saboteur.

Time and time again, I have seen people try to include an occasional glass of wine in their food plan and have watched their program gradually slide off the rails. I know giving up alcohol is tough for some people. If you find yourself balking, try letting it go for a trial period. It's worth it.

Bright Lines and When to Use Them

On Leap Day of 2012, I was nine years into my Bright Line journey and relaxing when my father-in-law, Hugh, tossed *The China Study* by T. Colin Campbell, Ph.D., and Thomas M. Campbell II, M.D., into my lap.[7] Once I started reading it, I couldn't put it down. The science it outlined on the cancer-causing effects of meat and dairy had such a profound effect on me that, for the rest of the weekend, I couldn't do much more than read the book and stare at the wall, processing what was on the page. I decided to stop eating meat and dairy that very day.

However, years later, I still don't have a personal Bright Line for meat and dairy. Why? Because my motivation for not eating meat and dairy is to maintain optimal health, not to rid myself of the obsession and compulsion that are the hallmark of addiction. If obsession and compulsion are the issue—smoking cigarettes, not being able to stop texting your toxic ex, self-harm—and you want to get past it, you need a Bright Line. If health is your objective, there is no evidence that perfect is better than "really good." Seriously. You can comply with a health goal 95 percent of the time, and it will benefit you as much as 100 percent perfection. That's another reason why hot dogs and Italian sausage are allowed on the Weight-Loss Food Plan, for example. And why I don't dictate that they be nitrate-free and organic, although, of course, that would be my suggestion.[8] If it takes eating a few things that feel decadent for you to get through the early days of adapting to Bright Line Eating, then knock yourself out. Like I said before, fine-tuning the health of your choices can come later.

Here's an example. A woman named Wendy Sax came to the Boot Camp a stubborn 40 pounds overweight. It drove her mad, mainly because she was vegan. From a nutritional standpoint, she thought she ate impeccably. But that weight still dogged her. What she learned through Bright Line Eating was that her quantities were much higher than they should have been. And she was eating sugar. And flour. And she grazed. Once she eliminated those things, she rapidly became Happy, Thin, and Free—not only from her excess weight, but from the mood swings that had plagued her for years.

Bright Line Eating works beautifully with other nutritional objectives you evolve over time—or bring with you to the program. But it has the power to permanently solve *weight* issues like nothing else.

One final note. Over time, we have developed an extensive FAQ database that covers everything, literally, from soup to nuts. What about tapioca? Coconut shavings? Aloe juice? There is not a question that has not been asked. Unfortunately, there isn't enough room here to include all those granular answers. We do have an extensive database for answering food questions on our website. Go to: http://ble.life/thebook, then click the Support button.

Case Study: Lois Boyd

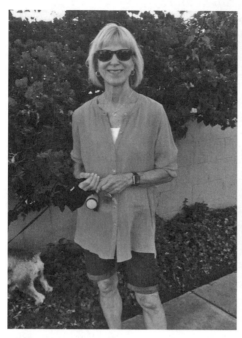 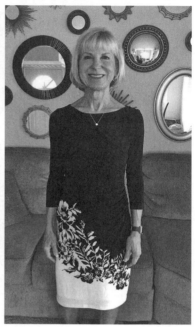

Highest Weight: 132 pounds
Current Weight: 103 pounds
Height: 5'2½"

My whole life, I had a huge secret: my relationship with food was out of control.

As in many families, there were always plenty of sweets in the house when I was growing up. Even though I had access to them at home, by the time I was a preteen, sugary treats had become so important to me that I would secretly find ways to get them.

In the mid-1960s, Twiggy emerged as a prominent teenage fashion model and thin was in. Although I was an average weight, I didn't feel thin enough, so I went on my first starvation diet. I dieted down to 106 pounds, and that's when my unhealthy relationship with food began.

I was unable to maintain a low-enough weight and started living in a black-and-white world of either rigidly following a diet or completely straying from whatever one I was on. I married at 21 and had my children at 22 and 25 years of age. After I had my kids, I was unable to return to my prepregnancy weight of 115 pounds. I turned to cigarettes, because I thought they would keep me thin. I smoked until my daughter started kindergarten and asked me to stop as part of an antismoking campaign at her school. My weight rose to 132 pounds. I turned to diet pills, diuretics, and laxatives to control my weight. I abused them for years and, at my worst, was taking 40 pills a day. Because I binged and abused laxatives, I was dehydrated, couldn't sleep, and had horrible cravings all the time.

In 2000, I dreamed of running a marathon, but that just isn't possible while taking laxatives. I found a doctor who helped wean me off them, enabling me to train. I placed third in my age group when I finally did run one, and running became my new passion.

My overall health continued to deteriorate due to my eating disorder, so I had to stop running. I was diagnosed with atherosclerosis in 2004. It was severe enough that my cardiologist wanted to treat my condition aggressively. I began taking several statins—until I found I couldn't tolerate them. My carotid arteries were getting more and more blocked due to my binge foods, and I desperately searched for a solution.

By that time my weight was normal—the same as it is today—I just couldn't stop the cycles of binging and restricting. In fact, I've been in a right-sized body for most of my life, as evidenced by my normal-looking "before" picture. Weight wasn't the problem—my insanity with food was.

I became a vegan in 2010, following the program of Dr. Joel Fuhrman. It was a wonderful plan, but I couldn't maintain it long-term. All it would take was a bite of "healthy" sugar, such as dried fruit, to trigger a binge. The bingeing became so severe that it would often leave me bedridden the following day and not back to normal for about four days. I felt totally out of control and broken. My health continued to decline. In addition to atherosclerosis, I also suffered from spinal stenosis, autoimmune conditions, osteoporosis, and gastrointestinal issues.

But then I discovered Bright Line Eating, in October of 2014, and my life completely changed.

Before Bright Line Eating my cholesterol was 193. Not awful, but my heart disease was advanced enough that my doctor wanted to get it under 150. When I started Bright Line Eating, it was hard to maintain my weight because my abused stomach couldn't handle the fibrous bulk of the vegetables and I was terrified of eating fat because of my heart disease and high cholesterol. Susan encouraged me to add some nuts to my plan to stabilize my weight. I was frightened, but I trusted her. I reluctantly agreed. Gradually my stomach issues cleared up and, within months, my cholesterol dropped to 131.

My cardiologist was—and still is—thrilled. After having check-ups every 4 months for 11 years, he now only wants to see me twice a year.

Across the board, my health is better. It took me nine months to regain my energy, but now I feel like a different person. My stomach issues are mostly gone. My sleep is better. But best of all, I'm not bingeing. Nothing could stop me—until I got the sugar and flour out of my system. When I was 103 pounds and eating vegan, I outwardly appeared to be a model of health, but when I was alone, I would often binge. I knew I was living a lie and I felt like a fraud.

Thanks to Bright Line Eating, I can finally be an authentic person. I am growing in ways I never imagined—like writing my story for this book. It's a huge step for me. Before Bright Line Eating, I told *no one* about my secret life with food. I was so embarrassed and ashamed. But I want others who struggle with food, even if they're in a normal-sized body, to know that Bright Line Eating can work for them. It's an amazing program. My happiness quotient has skyrocketed. I am finally *free*.

CHAPTER NINE

YOUR DAY 1: INTO ACTION

Welcome to the part of the book where you start taking action! If you have read every word up to this point, you are armed with all the information you need to understand how your brain has been blocking your weight loss and the food plan that can turn that around. Now it's time to take the steps to kick off your Bright Line Eating journey so your brain can heal. In this chapter, I am going to walk you through everything you need to do, step by step, before your first Bright Line day. And at the end of the chapter is a checklist that you can use to track your progress as you prepare.

Visit Your Doctor

This is the step that many people, in their understandable eagerness to get started, want to skip. I *highly* encourage you not to. First, if you are currently on any medications for medical conditions, it's very important to have your doctor's support and involvement before dramatically altering your diet. One thing I've seen over and over is that people's medications often need to be adjusted very quickly on this plan. Frequently, the need for medications is even eliminated since Bright Line Eating often resolves the myriad health issues that stem, ultimately, from the addiction to sugar and flour. What we have seen in our Boot Campers is that the scope of systemic healing is huge. Inflammation comes down, healthy gut flora proliferate, meal timing creates a fasting window that benefits the circadian rhythm of every organ, insulin and glucose systems balance, and cardiovascular damage reverses. This is not a promise, it's a prediction based on years of experience. So you'll want to ask your doctor what he or she thinks of you starting Bright Line Eating and then recruit supervision. You may want to make an action plan for how frequently you should check back in for potential medication adjustments.

Second, you want to get a full blood work-up. I suggest you get a full cholesterol panel, A1C, triglycerides, blood pressure, fasting blood glucose, baseline insulin reading, cbc test, and any other numbers that you and your doctor want to track. If you have had blood work done recently, you may feel comfortable skipping this step. But I highly recommend that you start off with a good benchmark, because things are about to change for you, rapidly and dramatically, and you can never get back that window into what your body is like now, at the beginning.

Take Your "Before" Pictures

If you have weight to lose, you'll want to take some good "before" pictures that show you at your current weight. Some people do this with eagerness and joy. Others will feel like I just suggested having a root canal without Novocaine. Please trust me on this one. Starting Bright Line Eating and not taking pictures of your "before" state is like raising a child without taking baby pictures. You'll never get this back. And this will work. And then no one will believe that you were ever fat, and you won't have proof. I am speaking from experience here. At my heaviest, I never allowed pictures to be taken. My best "before" picture, which you can see at http://ble.life/thebook, is NOT at my top weight. And I'm smiling in it. I would move heaven and earth now to have a picture of me with my big belly and all my bulges in their full glory, looking as miserable as I actually felt. At one point in my journey, I was a size 24. My best fat picture shows me at a size 14. Don't make that mistake. Please.

Another option is to shoot some video before you get started, and then keep capturing milestones of your journey as you proceed. What do you look like now, as you embark on this adventure? What does your fridge look like? What does your closet look like? How do you feel? Or be creative and capture your beginning in your own unique way. It doesn't have to be fancy or cumbersome—these days, any mobile device takes great videos.

Clean Out Your Kitchen

Donate, give away, or throw away everything that's not on your Food Plan. Check the refrigerator door for dressings, sauces, and condiments and clear out everything that has sugar, or any sweetener, listed in the first three ingredients.

Obviously, if you live alone, this step is much easier. If you live with others, clear out as much as you can while keeping things that your family or roommates will still want to eat. Depending on your circumstances, consider designating a refrigerator shelf and kitchen cupboard that will be only for your food. Or vice versa. Create a low or high shelf for others' food. Perhaps ask if you can pack all their snacks or sweets in a drawer or cupboard so you can simply avoid seeing them. However you do it, arrange your space to minimize triggers.

Things to Buy

I'm not a big "stuff" person. I don't need the latest or the greatest gadget, and I hate clutter. However, there are a few things I've learned you will need to make this journey successful. Think of it like climbing Everest: the right equipment will mean the difference between reaching the summit and sitting in a tent on a ledge. The list below will give you categories of what you'll need to buy, but for my latest recommendations on specific items I've found to work exceptionally well, please visit: http://ble.life /thebook.

1. Digital food scale. You don't need a fancy one with a calorie counter, nutrition information, or a printer—just a plain old food scale is all you need. But it must be digital. You don't want the ambiguity of trying to decide whether the needle is on the line, and you *definitely* don't want to be obsessing about how much lettuce you can smoosh into a measuring cup. Digital food scales are available at places like Target, Walmart, and Bed Bath & Beyond. You can also get them online. Features to look for: a pull-out display that will let you weigh your food in a large container or on a large plate (this is *so* helpful). Also get one that doesn't shut off automatically after one or two minutes. This allows you to chop salad vegetables and add them over time without having to start over because the scale shut off on you. The honest truth is that there is a HUGE difference between a good digital food scale and a not-so-good one. Trust me on this. I have a long-standing favorite that I've been recommending for years, but should a better one come out in the future, I'll post it on my website. To see my up-to-date opinions: http://ble.life /thebook.

2. Travel containers for food. Lightweight, plastic, semidisposable containers that come in packs of three or five work well. They have been redesigned to be safe for the microwave, dishwasher, and freezer. In particular, they do not contain the chemicals that are toxic in microwaves, but if you still don't feel comfortable microwaving food in plastic, buy plenty of glass or Pyrex containers, though they will be heavier in your lunch tote. If you want to keep something especially hot or cold, consider buying a thermal lunch bag as well.

Tip: For packing oil and vinegar for salad, search online for "sterile specimen cups." Yes, like the ones they have at your doctor's office. They're the perfect size, and they never leak!

3. Food journal. Consider buying a small, special journal to write your food in. If you go with a journal, you'll keep it in the kitchen by the fridge, with a pen.

4. Gratitude journal. Keep this by your bed to write in before you go to sleep. Again, I suggest buying one you find visually pleasing—it will encourage you to keep writing. If you want to see some journals I like, you can find them at http://ble.life/thebook in the "Tools" section.

5. Five-year journal. In 2010, I started writing in a five-year journal every night (yes, in addition to my gratitude journal) and I haven't missed a single night in all that time. I am in love with it. Here's how it works: there's a page for every day of the year, and there are five sections on each page. You are given a small handful of lines to encapsulate your day. After you've written for 365 days, you come back around to the beginning. Thereafter, you get to read what you wrote on that day the year before. And so on. It's a blast. And it's a perfect tool to pick up as you start a journey as momentous as Bright Line Eating. It's shockingly hard to find a good five-year journal these days, however. My favorite one is posted here: http://ble.life/thebook.

6. Bathroom scale. You'll want to make sure you have a good digital bathroom scale. An analog scale with a needle and an arc of numbers simply isn't a good choice these days. Toss it out, and go get yourself a digital bathroom scale. You'll want one that weighs by the half-pound, or perhaps in even smaller increments.

Social Support

Research shows that doing a weight-loss program with a friend or with social support increases your odds of success.[1] Recruit friends. You'll want to surround yourself with supportive people. It would be the *most* helpful to have them read Part I of this book, take the Food Freedom Quiz themselves, and talk about how their brain may work differently than yours. Even better would be to find some friends who want to travel on this journey with you. If there are no takers, no worries—you can find a thriving network in our Bright Line Eating Online Support Community: http://ble.life/thebook.

Picking Your Day 1

After you do the preliminary work, it's time to choose when your Day 1 will be. There are a few considerations here, and it's a balancing act. In some ways, there's never a good time—there will always be something looming on your calendar that you would usually think of as a "food occasion," be it a wedding, baby shower, or Thanksgiving. If you're going to stay Happy, Thin, and Free long-term, you'll need to have a program that can withstand holidays, cruises, and special occasions. I travel all the time and manage to stay within my Bright Lines. I celebrate birthdays and go to parties. I live out in the world, as do the thousands of successful people who have started this before you. We are not hermits. The power of this program is that you have clear rules to follow—and support to help you follow them.

So don't postpone starting, necessarily, just because a special event is coming up soon and you don't think you will be able to make it through. Note that my very first Boot Camp ever started in late October, so the first thing the participants were confronted with was Halloween, followed closely by Thanksgiving. And yet the Boot Camp was wildly successful. That said, you want to carve out space to do this well and be able to focus on it. So if you need to wrap up a few things in your life before starting, I totally get it.

The Last Ingredient

If your doctor is on board, you've taken your "before" pictures and videos, your digital food scale is out on the counter ready for action, and your social support network is lined up, then it's probably time to go grocery shopping and get the food you'll need for your first few days. Bring this book with you, and buy enough foods from each category of the Food Plan to get you through. You'll probably need more vegetables than you think, so buy those in large quantities. Also get some flash-frozen vegetables and some canned fruit—canned in juice, not syrup, of course—to have on hand as backup.

Your Checklist

1. Checkup
2. "Before" Photo
3. Clean Out Your Cupboards
4. Purchase:
   a. Digital Food Scale
   b. Travel Containers for Food
   c. Food Journal
   d. Gratitude Jornal
   e. Five-Year Journal
   f. Bathroom Scale
   g. Groceries
5. Social Support
6. Pick Your Day 1
7. Check http://ble.life/thebook to see if we've added any special tools you might want to use!

Day 1: Anatomy of a Successful Day

In many religions, such as Judaism and the Baha'i faith, the next day is thought to begin not at midnight, but at sunset. And so it is with Bright Line Eating. Your success on Day 1 is going to depend heavily on your preparations the evening before. Here's your mini-checklist:

1. Look in your fridge and decide what you're going to eat the next day.

2. Pick up the journal by the fridge and write "Day 1" at the top.

3. Write tomorrow's date.

4. Write down what you are committing to eat the next day.

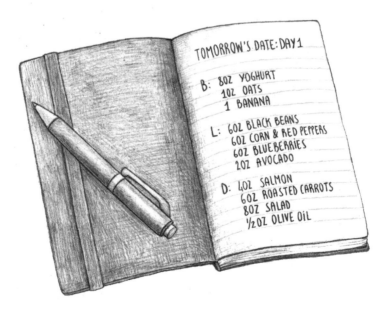

Get a good night's sleep. You are about to be rocketed into the fourth dimension.

In the morning on Day 1, you'll want to get your starting weight. Always weigh yourself first thing in the morning, naked, immediately after using the restroom.

How Often to Weigh?

There are three options for how often to weigh yourself. This is a deeply personal decision, with no right answer. Here are the pros and cons of each. See which sounds like the best fit for you.

Monthly: Many people who have used Bright Lines to lose their excess weight and keep it off for years strongly recommend that you only weigh yourself once a month while you're losing weight, transition to weighing once a week when you're within ten pounds of goal weight, and then continue weighing yourself weekly from there. The benefit of weighing once a month is that it encourages early freedom from the mind-chatter about your number. And it will help you avoid getting tripped up by the inevitable plateaus and fluctuations that will occur in your weight-loss journey. As the saying goes, "If you focus on your Bright Lines, you'll lose the weight. If you focus on the weight, you'll lose your Bright Lines." Most important, monthly weighing will take away the scale's power to determine your mood for the day. If you go with this option, I suggest that after your Day 1 weigh-in, you put your bathroom scale away somewhere—like in a closet. Then mark your calendar for the day you'll weigh yourself the following month. The downside is that you won't get short-term feedback on how much weight you're losing.

Daily: The second option is to weigh yourself every day. According to the National Weight Control Registry, this strategy is the most common among people who have lost weight and kept it off.[2] There is solid research to back up the efficacy of daily weighing. If you can stay emotionally detached from the number and stick to your food plan *no matter what the scale says* each morning, this option may work well for you. However, you'll have to make yourself mentally tough against the inevitable fluctuations. Pounds go up and down senselessly based on how long you've slept the night before, elimination and hydration levels, and normal hormonal activity for premenopausal women.[3] One stabilizing strategy, and one that I *strongly recommend* if you're going to weigh daily, is to graph your weight. Studies have shown[4] that seeing an image of your weight trend is an incredibly powerful tool for keeping commitments. It also helps you visualize that the slope is continuing to go down, even with speed bumps along the way.

That said, daily weighing may simply make you agitated, which is counterproductive. If you know yourself to be so attached to that number that it will derail your mood for the day to see your weight go up a bit, then don't weigh yourself every day. We want you thinking less about your weight, not more. In which case . . .

Weekly: This third option splits the difference. It combines the best of both worlds—you get some distance from the daily fluctuations on the scale that can mentally derail you if you are attached to what the number says, but you get the benefit of watching your progress unfold as your weight falls off. If you choose this last option, pick a specific day of the week for weighing yourself, and stick to it.

The Rest of Your Day 1

Think through your plan for the day and consider whether you'll need to pack and bring any of your meals with you. Better safe than sorry—if there's even the remote possibility that you may be out, bring your food. For example, if you're meeting with a friend for a long walk midmorning, but expect to be home by lunchtime, it's a good idea to think like a Boy Scout and "Be prepared." Pack your lunch. Remember silverware, a napkin, a sharp knife to cut your fruit if necessary, salt and pepper, and a nice big bottle of water.

On Day 1, your main focus will be on eating your precommitted three meals—and nothing in between. Weigh your food precisely. Six ounces of vegetables means 6.0, not 6.1 or 5.9. If that means you have to pinch off and remove half a green bean, then so be it. And remember the BLTs—no bites, licks, or tastes while you're cooking. No sneaking veggies from the cutting board into your mouth. Your first bite of food should be when you're sitting at the table and have taken a couple of deep breaths. Reflect for a moment on how good it feels to keep your commitment to yourself and eat exactly what you planned to eat. The purpose of this kind of precision is to build up integrity and credibility with *yourself*. If you've spent years, even decades, betraying yourself with food, it's just not worth it to switch your chicken for fresh fish at the last moment. You can have the fish tomorrow. It will be fine.

One Day at a Time

In a philosophical sense, you never truly get to decide what you're going to do on some future day. You never know whether you'll eat cake in a year. You can only decide whether you're going to eat cake right now. The question is not whether you will "have" to do this forever. You may wonder whether you will ever get to eat chocolate again, you will ever get to eat pizza again, whether you will get to eat cake at your granddaughter's wedding, and whether you will get to drink champagne on New Year's Eve. If this day is *not* New Year's Eve and it's *not* your granddaughter's wedding, you do not have that choice to make *right now*. Your choice right now is what are you eating and drinking *today*.

When I first got sober at 20, there was this old, crusty guy who used to say in the meetings, "I'm Jimmy, and I'm an alcoholic. I'm sober 35 years. I'm not going to take a drink today. I may very well drink tomorrow, but I'm not going to drink today." And I would think, "Why is he jinxing himself?"

I totally didn't get that *tomorrow never comes.*

So when someone asks me, "Do you ever get to have dessert again? How long are you going to do this for?" I just say, "I'm doing it today, and it seems to be working really well. I feel pretty great. So I'm going to keep doing it today. Beyond that, I have no idea."

The landscape of "today" is usually very comforting. Not always, but usually. Right here, right now, we're safe, we're fine. I always just come back to thinking, *What's my next meal? Can I picture eating that next meal? Can I picture eating the food I've committed to today?* Then I'm good. I don't have to decide today that I'm doing this forever.

As a matter of fact, I *never* have to decide that. I do this one day at a time.

Case Study: Julia Carol

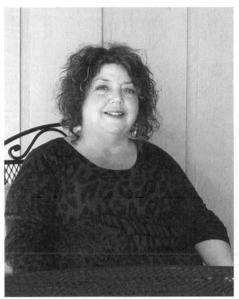 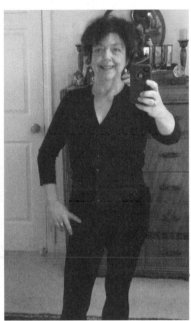

Highest Weight: 204 pounds
Current Weight: 122 pounds
Height: 5'2½"

While I wasn't overweight until I hit my teen years, I remember being super-focused on the acquisition of candy as a child. I'd even play with children I didn't enjoy all that much if their moms had bowls of candy out in their homes. In my teen years, my friends and I consumed copious amounts of junk food: candy bars, sodas, and all the fried foods and burgers we could get our hands on. I gained a lot of weight, and thus began my experiences with dieting.

I tried SlimFast, fasting, Jenny Craig, the grapefruit diet, and kept coming back to Weight Watchers after I'd failed at everything else. Sometimes I'd get as far as losing 10 or even 20 pounds . . .

only to find my willpower stretched so thin it would finally break and I'd gain back every pound, and then another 5 or 10.

In the 1980s, I found Living Thin Within and it led me to believe that moderation and listening to my body was the answer. But I couldn't seem to "stop when no longer hungry," which that plan calls for. I was always hungry.

I can't count how many dozens of times I joined Weight Watchers and a gym and vowed that THIS time I was going to get to goal. But over the years, even though my diet got healthier and I eliminated fast foods and most processed foods, ate more vegetables, and improved the quality of my sugar and flour products—premium organic ice cream and very expensive fair-trade chocolate and bakery breads and pastries—I still got fatter and fatter and fatter.

When I was 52, I was diagnosed as prediabetic. I already had tingling in my feet and stiffness in all my joints, hypertension (160/132), extremely high cholesterol (323 with the wrong HDL/LDL balance), high triglycerides, sleep apnea, insomnia, insulin resistance, and metabolic syndrome.

I felt such shame. I'd been able to change so many things in my life. I'd even been instrumental in changing smoking policy at the federal, state, and local levels. I'd helped clients change *their* lives and relationships . . . and yet I was a failure at helping my own body.

I continued to feel ashamed, hopeless, demoralized, frightened, old, stuck, and depressed about my health and my body until I saw Susan Peirce Thompson's *Food Freedom* videos. The information about leptin resistance and our dopamine receptors really made sense to me. And finding out that I'm a 10 on the Susceptibility Scale answered so many things. From the moment I started, I was determined to follow Bright Line Eating faithfully—a voice in my head told me to just obey the rules this time. My way hadn't worked.

The first few weeks on the program, I was like a deer in headlights. I walked into our co-op grocery and, though I thought I was a healthy shopper before, I suddenly wasn't sure what to buy or where to go. I was pretty nervous and terrified. I did have some cravings in the beginning, especially at night, but I just kept myself busy watching the videos in the Boot Camp modules. I wrote my food plan down faithfully every night before bed; I participated in the Facebook group; I got a buddy and a Mastermind Group fairly soon. I was on every coaching call. In short, I surrendered to Bright Line Eating in a way I'd never surrendered to anything before.

I began to release weight, and after about six weeks, I also saw significant other changes in my health. My blood pressure dropped dramatically. My fasting glucose rate came down to normal. I had energy. I slept through the night.

Here are my lab test results six months before starting BLE, and again a little over a year after starting BLE, after I'd been living at goal weight for several weeks:

6 months before starting BLE	14 months after starting BLE
Total cholesterol: 323	Total cholesterol: 155
Triglycerides: 299	Triglycerides: 85
LDL: 227	LDL: 99
HDL: 36	HDL: 39
Fasting glucose: 103	Fasting glucose: 85
Blood pressure: 160/132	Blood pressure: 96/64
Weight: 199	Weight: 122

I remember the joy I felt when I got back to the weight I'd been when I got married, when I weighed less than what it said on my driver's license, less than my husband, less than I ever had on any other diet. Now I'm at goal. I have never been here as an adult. Ever.

Now I love feeling my rib bones and hipbones when I lie in bed. I adore finding new clothes. Sometimes, I even need to go into the junior department because I'm so small. I fit nicely into airplane seats, don't snore, and feel about 30 years younger. But I'm humble enough to know that while I look thin, I am in recovery. I know who I am and I know what I am. I avoid unnecessary food cues and stay close to the Mothership. And I feel truly Happy, Thin, and FREE. My deepest wish is for others to find this program and achieve the success that I know can be theirs. I never thought in my wildest dreams that I would be a thin person helping others find success. I am forever grateful.

CHAPTER TEN

THE TOOLS THAT MAKE IT WORK

If a good food plan was all it took to achieve long-term weight-loss success, everyone would be thin already. It's not in the food plan. People don't believe that, but it's really, really not. What has led to success for thousands of Bright Line Eaters is a *comprehensive system* that sets up our lives so that we will stick with our food plan for months and years. The system supports and buttresses us at every turn. It keeps us on track. Again, the point here is to create automaticity and to keep inactive the parts of your brain that arouse your Saboteur. To make choosing foods that support and sustain your weight loss effortless and automatic. Eventually, you won't even notice you're doing it. It will be that ingrained.

Daily Rituals

The value of the daily rituals I'm going to suggest in the next few pages is that they help reinforce a Bright Line Life. If you are highly susceptible to the pull of refined foods, you have probably experienced the feeling of being out of control of the food that you put into your body for a long time. These rituals work in tandem with the food plan to put an end to that. They help heal your brain, reinvigorate your sense of control, and set you up for success. I strongly suggest you embrace these reinforcements. They play an integral role in your success on this journey.

Morning Routines

There are three rituals that I recommend you add to your morning routine. You might need to get up a little earlier to incorporate them. The first is making your bed. While that may seem obvious to many, when I suggest this in my Boot Camps, for many people it's an awakening. I don't know if it has to do with the sugar hangovers many people who come to Bright Line Eating have been living with for years, but for some reason we are a community that needs to be reminded to start making our beds. And when we do, it sets the day off on a positive foot. It's an act of respect for yourself and your home and it immediately says to your brain, "I am someone who accomplishes tasks. Go me!"

Inspirational Reading

For many, many years, I've carved out a small amount of time for inspirational reading in the morning. It started when I got sober and was told to sit quietly and read a daily meditation book every morning. In those days, my morning ritual consisted of a big cup of coffee with lots of cream and sugar sipped between puffs of cigarettes while I peacefully read the message for the day and sat with my Higher Power. It's come a long way since then, but those essential elements—minus the coffee and cigarettes—are still in play.

I must say here that Bright Line Eating is completely agnostic. It's not atheist. Just agnostic. So you can choose however much—or little—spirituality you want to infuse into your Bright Line Eating program. I'm very open about what I do, but I'm also emphatic that there is no requirement in Bright Line Eating that necessitates that anybody believe or do any specific things when it comes to spirituality or religion. That's all entirely up to you. I will share the science, however, which is that prayer and meditation replenish willpower.[1] That's just a fact.

On my website, you can find a list of daily readers I recommend: http://ble.life/thebook, but any kind of positive, uplifting daily meditation book will do. If you have a religious practice where you are enjoined by your faith to read some scripture morning and night, beautiful. I would encourage you to consider also adding a morning daily meditation reader that relates more specifically to your Bright Line Eating journey. If you connect to the ideas put forth here about food addiction, you might consider getting a daily reader that is specific to that. If you like poetry, you might consider getting a daily meditation reader by Rumi, who is one of the world's most beautiful epic poets. Essentially, anything works, so long as it will nourish you with positive thoughts to start your day.

Meditation

Meditation is incredibly valuable. Research shows that it keeps the brain young by slowing the atrophy of gray matter;[2] decreases activity in the default-mode network of the brain, resulting in increased happiness and decreased mind-wandering;[3] reduces depression, anxiety, and pain;[4] improves concentration and attention;[5] and can help alleviate addiction.[6]

You've probably heard about the enormous benefits of meditation. Yet you might find the thought of starting a regular meditation practice daunting. I know I did. For years upon years, I had a desire in the back of my mind to start meditating, but I procrastinated and put it off—until one of my mentors showed me a way of thinking about meditation that made it seem less scary. She told me that the key to meditating is to simply sit still. She said, "I don't care if you cross your legs or sit in a chair or sit on the couch or stand on your head, just don't *do* anything. No movement. No activity. No distractions. Nothing. For thirty minutes."

Finally, I was willing. She told me to set a timer and just sit there. So I did. And for many years, my meditation practice just consisted of quiet time. I didn't make any real effort to regulate what I was doing during those 30 minutes, other than keeping myself physically still.

The benefit that I got from setting aside that time, almost immediately, was a deep sense of comfort in my own skin. I can be at peace with myself even if I feel awful, if I feel sick, if I feel angry, if I feel really hungry, or if I'm having a food thought or a craving or an obsession. I can sit with those feelings and just let them *be*. And that is something I most definitely could not do in 2003 when I first started to meditate.

The benefit of just sitting in stillness is developing a little bit of a pause between the stimuli in your environment and your response to them. Ideally, there's a nice pause there. And in that pause you get to *choose* your response, as opposed to just reacting. Trust me, it's a life changer.

A word about posture. I'm personally not flexible enough to meditate lotus style. I have chronic back issues, and even sitting cross-legged for several minutes really hurts my upper back, so for years I sat in a chair. But after my twins were born, I found that, with my body fully supported in the chair, I would just fall asleep. To my credit, I stayed faithful to my daily practice, show-ing up each morning to sleep in that chair. It was so predictable that I'd even factor it into my calculations at night: "Let's see, I'm turning out the lights at 10:00 P.M., and my alarm is set for 5:00 A.M., so I'm getting seven hours of sleep tonight, but I'll get thirty minutes more during meditation tomorrow morning, so that's seven and a half." I tried tinkering with my setup by using various chairs and different approaches, but no matter what I changed, I'd still wind up asleep in my morning meditation.

Until I found a meditation bench.

I *love* my meditation bench! It's a padded, tilted bench that sits low to the ground and supports your weight as you kneel on the floor. It makes my back feel wonderful because it tilts my pelvis at just the right angle so that my spine rests in the perfect curvature atop my sitting bones. Mine has folding legs so I can travel with it. And travel with it I do. Total game changer. I haven't fallen asleep in my morning meditation in *years*.

Regarding breathing, I don't usually force myself to do much by way of breathing exercises, but I'm open to that and I encourage you to explore whatever meditation apps or soundtracks or breathing practices or mantras work for you. If you're new to meditation, there are many great resources online. At http://ble.life/thebook, I list several that people in the Bright Line Community have found easy and enjoyable. There are a million ways to meditate and, as far as I'm concerned, they're all legitimate paths up the mountain. If, after reading this section, you still feel apprehensive about starting a meditation practice, definitely check out this website and pick an easy getting-started training program. There are very, very painless ways to begin, and it's more than worth the effort.

You also don't have to start by going for 30 minutes. If 30 minutes sounds impossible, start with a window of time that seems really doable, even if it's two minutes, and build up from there. If you meditate for two minutes tomorrow morning and add one minute every day after that, you'll be up to 30 minutes within a month. And 30 minutes doesn't have to be the goal. Research shows that even 10 to 15 minutes of regular meditation confers huge benefits.[7]

I also want to acknowledge that nobody's morning has extra minutes in it. The key to meditating in the morning is to set your alarm earlier. The good news is that Bright Line Eating makes it easier to get up earlier because you're not fueling your body after dinner. You will naturally fall asleep earlier than you do now and wake up *far* more refreshed than you're used to. Within this new environment, carving out a few minutes in the morning to meditate will be easier than you think.

And, you know, I'm not the Bright Line Eating police. So I'm not going to knock on your door and say, "Hey, are you meditating?" It's your journey, but meditation will pay huge dividends in your Bright Line Eating practice because it will give you a way to regulate your emotions and thoughts before you run to food for comfort. It's a respite.

Committing Your Food

In the last chapter, we talked about the importance of writing down the night before exactly what you plan to eat the next day and then sticking to it precisely. I want to take it a step further now. I want to encourage you to *commit* what you're going to eat for the day. This is not the same as merely writing it down. Writing it down in your journal marks your decision; a commitment will help you stick to that decision.

Committing your food is one of the key components of Bright Line Eating that takes the load off of willpower. Many studies have verified that a verbal or public commitment of some specific action that you're planning to take is an incredibly effective way to bolster willpower and increase success.[8] It works, and it's an invaluable habit to build.

You can do it in the evening, right after you write down your food for the next day, or you can do it the following morning before your day gets going. Whichever you pick, always do it the same way consistently. Again, we're building *habits* to take the load off willpower.

Let's talk about the different ways you can do this.

1. The first option is to make the commitment inside the Bright Line Eating Online Support Community. There you'll find a group of like-minded people traveling with you on this journey. One of the benefits of committing your food in the Online Support Community is that it will always be there for you. It's not going to miss your phone call. It's not going to leave the program. It's there for you in perpetuity. So you can rely on it, always, as a platform for committing your food. For that reason,

I think it's a really great option. Find us at http://
ble.life/thebook.

2. The second way is to commit it live, by telling
    another human being. The benefit of this method
    is that you know there's a specific individual who is
    party to the commitment, and to whom you will be
    accountable. It will feel great to tell them the next
    day that you stuck to your commitment. It's a very
    powerful sort of contract.

3. The third way to commit your food is to yourself
    or to God and to have a ritual around how you
    do that. If you're a person of faith, you could get
    on your knees and read your food plan out loud
    and say, "God, I commit to eat only and exactly
    this food and nothing else tomorrow." If you're
    someone who, instead, has faith in the highest
    manifestation of your best self, you could do the
    same thing. You could read your food plan out
    loud and say, "I commit to my Highest Self that
    I will eat only and exactly this tomorrow." The
    only downside of committing to yourself or to
    God is that it's less public. And research shows
    that committing things publicly, either to another
    human being or to a community forum, like
    our Online Support Community, is really, really
    effective.[9] So I encourage you to choose whichever
    feels more intuitive for you and stick to it. Again,
    consistency is key.

Finally, I would suggest that you not use multiple methods.
Sticking with one method is best. The reason is this: if you commit your food by telling a buddy *and* you post it online, then
if one day you only manage to commit to one of those places,
you might feel half-committed. You don't want to put yourself
in that situation.

I myself committed my food every single day for the first couple of years that I did Bright Line Eating. I don't do it anymore. And what you'll find is that, most likely, you won't need to do it forever. But be careful thinking that you're there too soon. It took me years to get to a place where I could trust myself to stick with my food plan, day in and day out, without making that commitment. Not months—years. So I encourage you to find a way to commit your food, start doing it, make it a habit, and watch what happens. It's going to serve you really well.

Evening Routine

The most important evening routine you should institute when you begin Bright Line Eating is to write down your food for the next day in your little food journal next to the fridge. Do it immediately after dinner. Then, if you are an evening committer, commit your food for the following day. After you do, you'll relax, knowing the bulk of the next day is taken care of. Your only task for the next day will be to eat only and exactly what you've written down. That's it. No decisions to make in the moment, no negotiations when you're tired and vulnerable to the Willpower Gap, just one commitment to eat what you chose when you were relaxed and full.

Then, once you get into bed but before you turn out the light, pick up your gratitude journal and reflect on the day a bit. If you've never kept a gratitude journal, I recommend you start with an exercise called "Three Good Things." The way it works is simple: each night, write down three things that went well that day and a bit about *why* they went well. This exercise is simple but incredibly powerful. It works because it changes your focus. We are so quick to notice what goes wrong in our lives— an adaptive behavior that helped us survive before we secured our place at the top of the food chain. But today, dwelling on the negative can create a lot of unhappiness. Dr. Martin Seligman, professor of psychology at the University of Pennsylvania and author of *Flourish*, as well as many other titles, explains:

> People who are grateful tend to be happier, healthier and more fulfilled. Being grateful can help people cope with stress and can even have a beneficial effect on heart rate. In tests, people who tried it each night for just one week were happier and less depressed one month, three months and six months later.[10]

The three things do not have to be big. They could be something as simple as: "I weighed and measured my breakfast. I found it to be really delicious. It was enough."

Then explore *why* it went well—why did weighing and measuring your food and having a filling Bright Line breakfast occur? Well, perhaps because you carved out the time to weigh and measure your food and you realize you are finally taking care of yourself. Or it might be that it felt like enough for the first time today because your body is acclimating as the result of the good actions that you took yesterday and the day before. That's what I mean by *why*. What explains how that good thing came to pass? What have you done, now or in the past, or what has someone else done, now or in the past, that resulted in that good thing you wrote down manifesting in your life?

The next step is to encapsulate your day in the five-year journal. You only have a handful of lines to write, so it won't take long. But trust me, watching your life unfold, day after day, year after year, is an incredibly valuable and satisfying practice.

You might want to close out your day with another spiritual or inspirational reading to put your mind in a good place before sleep, but that's optional.

The Nightly Checklist Sheet

Bright Line Eating involves breaking a suite of long-standing habits and replacing them with a more effectual set of new habits. The way we establish, monitor, and cement this new lifestyle is with our Nightly Checklist Sheet. It lists the behaviors, from writing our food down the night before to making our bed in the morning to making our gratitude list, that are part and parcel of living Happy, Thin, and Free forever. I've included a sample Nightly Checklist Sheet at the back of the book, and on my website you can also download a template to make your own. I'm fully expecting you to modify it because this is a living, breathing, fluid document that should be customized for each person, and will even differ for individuals from month to month. I change mine typically every three weeks at least. This template is simply a suggestion and a starting point.

The reason to make changes in your Nightly Checklist Sheet is to make sure it accurately reflects what you truly feel committed to and the areas you want to monitor. So having something on there that you wish you were doing in theory but aren't actually doing is hugely counterproductive.

In my experience, people stop doing the Nightly Checklist Sheet because they use it the wrong way. It shouldn't reflect what you think you SHOULD be doing, or what you WISH you were doing, it should show what you ARE committed to doing, right now, as evidenced by your actions. If all you're really doing is writing down your food the night before, sticking with your Bright Lines each day, and walking your dog, then you have three things on your checklist. And that's totally fine. The minute your soul cries, *"But wait! I want to be doing a gratitude list each night!"* Then that should go on your Nightly Checklist Sheet as well. It will grow and change. Modify it often.

You may also need to customize the line about weighing yourself. If you're weighing yourself weekly and not daily, then on your weekly weigh day it might say, "I weighed myself once and exactly once today. Here was my weight. Here was the change from last week." For every other day, state, "I surrendered my weight today and did not hop on the scale."

Toward the end of the Nightly Checklist Sheet, you'll see an item about getting enough sleep. Again, if seven or eight hours isn't the amount of sleep you need, change that, or if getting enough sleep isn't really something you think you need to remind yourself to do, take it off. I want you to make it work for you and reflect what you are committed to doing.

When you use the Nightly Checklist Sheet regularly, it will serve as a powerful tool to help you achieve new things that matter to you in your life. Let me give you an example. Several years ago I got two speeding tickets back to back, which was incredibly expensive and embarrassing. I considered myself a pretty responsible, together person, and to have been ticketed twice by the same cop going 90 miles an hour was mortifying.

On my Nightly Checklist Sheet, I added "I did not drive more than five miles over the speed limit today." And I kept it there until driving slowly and sanely became an ingrained habit. Now it's no longer on the list.

I encourage you to buy a clipboard for your current Nightly Checklist Sheet and keep it by your bed, either on your bedside table or inside your bedside drawer. Develop the habit of noting all the habitual behaviors you completed during the day before you turn in. Research shows we will do more of the things we want to do more often if we are monitoring and seeing, in black and white, whether or not we have done them.[11]

When I'm going over my Nightly Checklist, I check the box for everything I've done that day. If I haven't done something, I circle the entire square. At a glance, I can tell if my week is staying on track with my Bright Line Eating journey.

The Emergency Action Plan

The Emergency Action Plan (EAP) is a set of tools for you to use in dire situations. It is not a substitute for developing good habits—what I call "if/then" habits. For example, *if* I'm out and about and the urge to eat what other people are eating is creeping up on me, *then* I excuse myself to go to the restroom and activate my Emergency Action Plan. You'll need it, especially at first, because the urge to eat foods that are not included in your plan is likely to come up. Maybe every hour, maybe every day, maybe only once in a while. But even if it's every nanosecond—don't worry, we've got you.

There are five things that research shows will really help you resist temptation in the moment. They replenish willpower and get you right back on track.

1. Social Support. The first and most effective tool is human connection.[12] So if you have a friend or a support buddy that you can call or text, that is the best thing. Human connection is also available within our Bright Line Eating Online Support Community. You can always post something really quickly in a restaurant or at a party. It doesn't have to be long to be effective—just a quick, honest message asking for help: "Hey, I'm really struggling here. At a party. The food is calling to me, but I commit to you all that I'm not going to eat any of it." You can send out a post like that and just know that love and support is pouring your way. And when you get home at the end of the night, you can read all the comments and supportive messages others have posted in return. It's such a great way to feel connected.

In my Bright Line Eating journey, social support has been *the* single most effective tool for keeping me on track. But I'm an extreme extrovert and a 10 on the Susceptibility Scale. You may find that you can manage without hundreds of people having your back at every moment. Find the level of support that works for you. Having more is generally better. Use it all. Really, really use it. Make it a habit to post in the Online Support Community, or text or call a friend when cravings strike. Some folks in Bright Line Eating have credited the support available in our online community as the number-one factor that contributed to their success. You are not alone in this. There are literally thousands of people walking this path along with you. Join us.

2. Prayer. The second research-verified method for replenishing willpower in the moment is prayer.[13] So if you're a praying person, this is good news to you. Pray. Pray. Pray. Remove yourself from the situation and go to the bathroom. Go wherever you can take a moment away and ask God to relieve your temptation to eat. Ask God to give you strength. Say a favorite prayer. Sit for a moment, and just ask for help. Then watch as you get through the rest of the day without deviating from your food plan. It is so powerful.

3. Meditation. If you're at a party or a restaurant, you can always excuse yourself to go to the bathroom. Sit in there, take some deep breaths, and just quiet your mind and your body down for a bit. Just five minutes of meditation is enough to replenish your willpower.[14]

4. Gratitude. No matter where you are in the world, no matter at what party or occasion, no matter what restaurant, you can always turn your mind toward gratitude. You can jot down a quick Gratitude List on the back of a receipt. You can type it into your smartphone. You can do it silently in your head. You can whisper it to a friend. It's amazing how turning your thoughts to gratitude will ease those temptations.[15]

5. Service. Last, when you stop thinking of yourself and focus on others, it's easier to stop obsessing over things that only relate to you. Get into service. Addictive eating is an isolating, insular, self-absorbed, mind-numbing phenomenon.[16] Service dispels all of that. The definition of "service" can run the gamut of doing something nice or helpful for someone else, from giving a compliment or a smile to joining a service-based organization in your area. In the moment, at a restaurant or party, you can turn to the person next to you, or look for someone who is alone, and strike up a conversation with them. Play with kids. Clear plates. Ask questions. Be interested in others. Be *present* for them.

For over a decade, my service was to help people in my community discover and follow this way of eating. Every morning at 5:30 A.M., after my morning meditation, I would take phone calls—15 minutes per call, back-to-back—from the people who had asked me for help. I would guide them in their weight-loss journey and listen to their food commitments for the day. This service helped them, but I believe it helped me at least as much. It allowed me to start each day flooded with gratitude and feeling connected. It also reminded me that, despite the dark times and challenges I have faced, I am a USEFUL person. Rebuilding that sense of confidence and purpose as you shed your excess weight is invaluable. So look around your community—I am sure it is full of need. See where what you have to offer can fit.

So. Human connection, prayer, meditation, gratitude, and service bring us to five strategies for avoiding temptation during emergencies. There's also a sixth strategy that's infinitely adaptable: *distraction*. Go for a walk, take a bath, knit, or do a puzzle. Some people also find that when they want to eat, just prepping their healthy food for the next day can be very comforting. Other people need to stay out of the kitchen. What you choose is up to you, but find a way to distract yourself. Maybe brushing and flossing your teeth is a good idea. Often when we've brushed our teeth and rinsed with some mouthwash, that residual minty taste in our mouth makes us not want to eat anymore. It's a good trick. Figure out, in advance, a list of things that could serve to distract you from thoughts about eating.

Last, I encourage you to write down your Emergency Action Plan, with the steps you plan to follow, in order. Start it at the top by saying, "Before I deviate from my food plan, I commit to taking the following actions." Make sure there are at least five things on there that you will really commit to doing, and keep that piece of paper with you at all times.

Mastermind Groups and Buddies

A Mastermind Group is a small group, ideally four people, who come together on a weekly basis to support each other, brainstorm, hold each other accountable, and grow together in their Bright Line Eating journey. I believe the Mastermind Group concept was first popularized in Napoleon Hill's classic book *Think and Grow Rich*, first published in 1937.[17] Since then, Mastermind Groups have become very popular, particularly in the business world.

When I left my 12-Step food addiction program some time ago, I instantly knew that, without live meetings, sponsorship, and accountability, I'd be at risk of having my addictions flare back up. So I formed a Mastermind Group. We call ourselves the Magnificent Mavens Mastermind Group, and we meet once a week for 90 minutes, on the phone, using a free teleconference line. (There are many conferencing services that are free and easy to use. For my current recommendation, go to http://ble.life/thebook.) Each of us gets an allotted amount of time to share, get support, and get feedback. I'm including the structure of our weekly call here. The Mastermind call isn't a time to chitchat. Its value will be increased tenfold if you adopt this structure, or one similar, and stick to it.

Mastermind Call Structure (90 minutes; 4 people)

1. Welcome each other. (4 minutes)

2. Facilitator asks who wants to go first, second, third, and fourth that day. (1 minute)

3. Opening round: facilitator asks each person to complete the following: (10 minutes)

   - Right now I'm feeling _____.

   - My "win" for the past week was _____.

   - Regarding my commitment from last week,
     I _____.

4. Facilitator sets a timer for 16 minutes, and the first person uses that time to share how they are feeling, discuss any struggles or challenges they're having, and get support from the other people in the group. Sharing for 10 minutes and leaving 6 minutes to get feedback and support is a good practice. When the timer goes off, it's the next person's turn. (64 minutes)

5. Closing round: facilitator asks each person to complete the following: (8 minutes)

   - My "takeaway" from this week's call is

     _____.

   - This week I commit to _____.
     (One person writes down these commitments in a safe place so they can be referenced the following week. People will forget.)

6. Scheduling. Make sure everyone can attend at the usual meeting time next week, find an alternative time if not, and pick a facilitator for the following week. (3 minutes)

We still meet weekly, to this day, and we are incredibly committed to supporting each other on this journey. My Mavens enrich my life immeasurably. I can't recommend a Mastermind Group strongly enough. If you can drum up three other people who are as committed to this way of life as you are, you will find yourself supported and buoyed every step of the way. It's priceless.

If you can't find three participants, get yourself just one person to support you—we call this having a "buddy." Your buddy is someone you can commit your food to and call on in an emergency. Many people in Bright Line Eating find that having a Mastermind Group *and* a buddy, or even two or three buddies, is the way to go. The more support, the better.

If you can't find anyone in your neighborhood who's also doing Bright Line Eating, please visit our website and consider joining a Bright Line Eating Boot Camp and joining our community online—it's also a great place to find people to join you in forming a Mastermind Group. You might consider stating where you are on the Susceptibility Scale, if you have a preferred time zone, day, or time, and if you want to be in a mixed-gender or same-sex group. And if and when you create that group, I think you will find, as I have, that it provides a framework and environment for growth in your Bright Line Eating journey that can't be surpassed by any other.

In particular, if you're struggling with your Bright Line Eating journey, the Mastermind Group provides a solid structure that can provide the support you need to get back on track—and stay there. And if you're not struggling, I encourage you to throw out a lifeline to one or two people who are. It's a way we lift each other up as a community.

I strongly encourage you to incorporate these tools into your life starting from Day 1—they are as much a part of Bright Line Eating as the Food Plan and the Bright Lines themselves. I promise they will make the difference between losing your excess weight and silencing your Saboteur . . . or not.

I know they will work for you if you use them.

Case Study: Teresa Stawicki

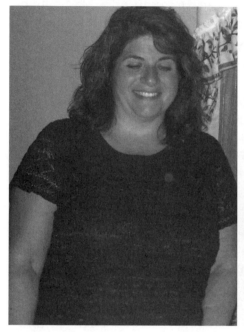 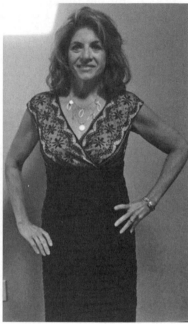

Highest Weight: 230 pounds
Current Weight: 125 pounds
Height: 5'2"

I'm from an Italian family. We related and connected to each other through pasta. You couldn't come by to drop a package off at our house without my mom offering to feed you. Eating was encouraged when I was a kid, but by age 12 I remember being told that I couldn't just eat as much as I wanted to. All of a sudden, it seemed, my dad started telling me, "You shouldn't eat so much." My mom was overweight, so I think my dad was probably trying to protect me from getting as heavy as she was. Of course, when they started trying to control my portions I started looking for food elsewhere.

I started eating outside the home. If I had a few extra dollars, I'd spend it on a treat for myself, in private. We didn't have a lot of money so we weren't given a whole lot of extras growing up, which meant that going to a fast-food place seemed like a real luxury. Or I'd sneak something from the vending machine at school. I was always trying to hide food.

When I was 14, I first started trying to lose weight. I weighed about 148 pounds. I got a diet book and tried to follow it. I didn't even fully understand all of it, but I did lose 10 pounds. Of course as soon as I lost that weight I gave up on it and went back to my usual ways.

Then I tried Weight Watchers at 18. I went on and off it a few times, even managing to get down to 128 pounds when I was trying to attract my first boyfriend. But once I landed him, I stopped trying. We got married, I relaxed my habits, and the next thing I knew I had plumped up to 170 pounds. So I rejoined Weight Watchers. I got down to 134 pounds. But I could never stay at my weight without being on a diet. Every time I lost weight, I'd go back up—plus another 10.

In my head I could hear my mother saying, "If you're not thin, no one's going to like you." I thought the weight made me who I was.

When I was 27, I got pregnant with my oldest daughter. I was afraid of getting any fatter, so I tried to stay on Weight Watchers throughout the pregnancy. But then I got pregnant again five months later. I had two babies at home, a new house, so I stayed in and *ate*. By my second daughter's second birthday, I weighed 230 pounds. I was 30.

I joined Weight Watchers *again*. I only lost about 26 pounds—because, of course, I saved all my points for desserts. Every time I allowed sweets to come into the program, my mentality would shift from dieting to hopelessness and it would be over.

Three years later, I joined again. But I wasn't losing. I was eating sugar. I was eating flour. I could never stay true. I gained it all back.

In my early forties, I started exercising. But all *that* did was give me "permission" to keep eating. I maintained a weight between 205 and 215 for about six years. I couldn't seem to get below 200. Then, in 2014, I tried Dr. Jonny Bowden's program and lost 24 pounds . . . but then I went on a cruise vacation and by the end I was eating full portions of dessert again. I started gaining it back. I just felt so hopeless.

Then I found Bright Line Eating. Once I understood that sugar was working like a drug on my brain, honestly, everything was smooth sailing.

My biggest challenge was social situations. In my Italian community, I'd have to defend myself and keep saying, "No thank you, that's not how I eat anymore." I'd have to get belligerent at times because people kept saying, "Oh, just have a little cake. It won't hurt you." Before Bright Line Eating, I would have given in. But now I knew even one bite would hurt me very much. I had to be very direct with my mother and father in particular. But when they finally saw how I was losing weight, they began to understand and started supporting me. In fact, my mother joined me—and now she's lost 25 pounds! Her health has also improved dramatically.

My life now is beautiful. I feel in control and very, very energetic. I'm happy with myself. I'm really a different person. I don't have any more aches and pains in my knees and heels. My cholesterol numbers are fabulous. My resting heart rate is better. My blood pressure is low.

Best of all, the weight loss has given me so much more confidence. I'm not afraid anymore. I even enrolled in a course and have become a certified life coach. Once I got clearheaded, I realized that I have a lot to give. I want to help people. Bright Line Eating has changed my life.

Part IV

THE ROAD MAP: STAYING ON COURSE

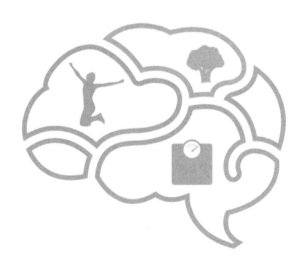

CHAPTER ELEVEN

BRIGHT LINE LIVING

Bright Line Eating creates sustainable weight loss because it isn't some crash diet; it's a lifetime weight-loss solution. And a lot of things come up over the course of a lifetime. Things that used to involve eating, for happy reasons or sad. I want to equip you with as much information as I can about how to navigate a full and rich life while staying fully Happy, Thin, and Free. I want Bright Line Eating to be sustainable and joyful for you. I don't want you to EVER regain your weight. Your happiness is too precious to me. Truly.

So in these next three chapters, we're going to cover the most common things that could crop up and threaten to throw you off your game. I'm going to offer some suggestions on how to handle them. I can't go into as much detail here as I do in the Boot Camp, because that would take volumes, but you will get the essentials.

What to Expect in the Weight-Loss Phase

We touched on this a little bit in Chapter Nine, but the reality is that, physiologically speaking, losing weight is pretty hard on the body, for several reasons. First, we don't gain or eliminate fat cells—the ones we've got just expand and contract as our weight fluctuates. When fat cells shrink, it has big implications for how we feel because fat cells, it turns out, are the landfills, the storage dumps of the body. They store toxins of all sorts, sometimes, literally, for *years*.[1]

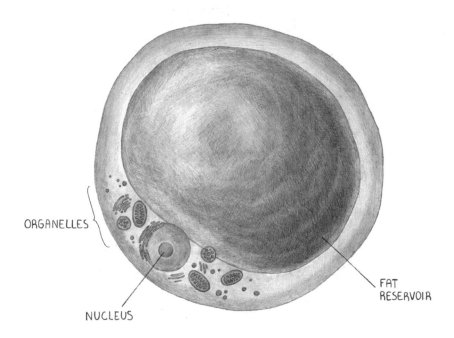

ORGANELLES

NUCLEUS

FAT
RESERVOIR

See that massive fat reservoir in the picture of the fat cell? Well, it doesn't just contain fat. It's also a storage space for toxins. When you shrink your fat cells, what do those reservoirs do? Well, they migrate over to the cell membrane and dump their contents into the bloodstream.[2] The fat gets burned for fuel, and the toxins get processed by the liver. All day, every day. Toxins, toxins, toxins. So drink a lot of water to help flush those toxins. And expect to feel *tired*. Also note that you'll be getting a lot of your fuel now from your stored fat, which is not the body's preferred fuel source. Yet another reason you won't feel in peak form during these brief weight-loss months.

Part of the tiredness will also come from not eating enough calories to sustain your metabolic needs, but this is why we lose weight. Expect that your metabolism will slow down to somewhere between 70 and 90 percent of its typical functioning.[3] One of the mechanisms for this metabolic slowdown is a decrease in thyroid hormone, which is the hormone that stokes your metabolic engine. On blood tests, this can look like hypothyroidism. And, in a way, it is. But it's *temporary* hypothyroidism induced by decreased caloric intake—it's what your body *wants* to be doing, so there's no need to medicate it away. It will reverse naturally when you transition to the maintenance phase and start eating more food again. This is all the body's natural response to weight loss. Make no mistake, losing weight is stressful on the body. But we've got you on a food plan that's going to allow you to keep losing weight for the long term, without feeling excessively hungry.

You might be wondering, "Should I be overly concerned about this? Will my metabolism rebound?" It's true that there is research that argues that it won't, including a now-famous study showing that graduates of *The Biggest Loser* have metabolisms that never recovered from the extreme calorie depravation they were put through.[4] It's important to say we have never seen evidence of this happening in Bright Line Eating. After getting down to goal weight and transitioning to maintenance, people are able to eat a surprisingly large amount of food with few cravings and typically little to no hunger. So, no, I don't think there's reason for alarm. In the long run, losing the weight is the very best thing you can do for your health. The negative side effects of weight loss are all temporary.

I believe that another reason we feel tired in the early days of Bright Line Eating is that most of us have been habitually using caffeine and sugar to push past our natural limits, to give ourselves that extra pick-me-up. When we can't do that anymore, we can feel like we're hitting a wall. The body finally starts to demand the rest it has been needing for a very long time.

So if you're tired, *rest*. If you can't rest, at least travel gently. This is where, like I said in Chapter Seven, I suggest you imagine you're wearing bunny slippers. That's the kind of attitude I want you to take toward this early weight-loss phase, because it's exhausting—but it's temporary. In general, in my experience after coaching thousands of people, it goes away by Day 90. Sometimes it lasts longer, but oftentimes it ends well before that. Also, it's true that some people skip the tired phase altogether and begin to feel fantastic as soon they start Bright Line Eating. But, either way, eventually Bright Line Eating results in abundant, overflowing energy—with no dips—all day long. So hunker down, keep your eye on the ball, and be patient with the process.

What to Say to People About Your Weight Loss

Your body is going to start changing, and people may begin to ask you about it. It might feel sort of nosy or intrusive, but people don't mean any harm. They are just interested and curious. Your response is really up to you. I always told everyone what I was doing and why, but I'm pretty open. If someone's asking you pointedly *why* you're not eating this or that and you really don't want to get into it with them, you could simply say, "I just found out I have food allergies and sensitivities." This is very true. To say I'm *sensitive* to sugar and flour is an understatement. When I ingest sugar and flour, I break out in obsession, cravings, and obesity. In my book, that's an allergic reaction.

I also happen to have experienced abstaining from sugar and flour for long periods of time and then ingesting them again and having really dramatic reactions (e.g., flu-like symptoms, hives, headaches, and other physiological effects). So I now really do believe that I am allergic to sugar and flour. They do not agree with me. But whether it's a metaphor or a physiological reality, either way it's helpful. It's helpful to say, "I've discovered I have food allergies and sensitivities. I've stopped eating sugar and flour, and I find that it's really working for me."

Or, if you have any other conditions—arthritis or migraines or insomnia—that you find that Bright Line Eating has alleviated, you can always fall back on those. Try saying, "I experimented with eliminating sugar and flour from my diet and my headaches have gotten a lot better, so now I'm not eating them anymore."

The main thing to keep in mind is that nobody cares that much. People are not focused on you; they are focused on themselves. I want to propose something else: If somebody seems really interested, it's probably because they have a food issue themselves. Take the opportunity to be helpful to them. Share the road map out of the misery and hell of overeating. Even if all you say is, "I've stopped eating sugar and flour," you will have planted a seed that later might grow into something beautiful.

Cooking for a Family and the Division of Responsibility

This is a topic that's dear to my heart because I have three daughters. It's also something I know a lot about because, for many years, I taught a college course on the psychology of eating, and in that course I included a unit on the psychology of feeding kids. My go-to reference in this domain is a nutritionist named Ellyn Satter.* She has a philosophy on food that is very different than Bright Line Eating, so brace yourself if you decide to look her up. She does not believe in food addiction at all. She believes in being what she calls a "competent eater,"[5] which means giving yourself permission to eat as much as you want of whatever you want, in a focused and attentive way, when it's mealtime. If you're overweight, she suggests not worrying about it. She and I have talked, and have agreed to disagree on this. Competent eating never worked for me, and I believe there are people with highly susceptible brains who will find it doesn't work for them, either. For people who are low on the Susceptibility Scale, it may work great. That said, I *do* recommend her approach to feeding kids. While I am aware that thousands of children in the United States are overweight or obese, kids are not grown-ups, so I think it's wrong to steer them, even subtly, into Bright Line Eating.

---

*   See: http://ellynsatterinstitute.org/other/ellynsatter.php.

Bright Line Eating is a choice people must make on their own. It's a program for people who *want* it, not for people who *need* it.

But we want to help our kids be healthy eaters. We do. So, what can we do? Well, one of the best things we can do when we're feeding kids is stick to structured meals. If you're a parent who is adopting Bright Line Eating, that is wonderful—you're going to be instituting breakfast, lunch, and dinner with a regularity that you might never have done before, and that's going to be a good thing for the kids in your life.

A key idea of Satter's that I think is essential—and that has saved my own sanity when it comes to feeding my kids—is something she calls the "division of responsibility."* This clearly delineates what *my* job is and what *their* job is when it comes to food.

The job of the parent is to decide when the meal is happening, where it's happening, and what's being served. When, where, and what. But, as soon as the food is on the table, *the parent's job ends*. Then the child's job is to decide, on his or her own, how much, if any to eat of what's being served.

I was very lucky that I learned about the division of responsibility when my firstborns—twin girls—were still infants. I have never in my life pressured my kids to eat anything. Ever. They don't have to eat their vegetables before they can get a bite of whatever they consider the "good stuff" or before they can leave the table. They don't have to try at least one bite of everything. They don't have to finish what's on their plate. As soon as I've provided the meal, I become blind, deaf, and dumb. I don't even pay attention to what they choose or refuse.

What this means is that if part of what I'm serving is starch and all they want to eat is rice with butter on it, they can eat that. They can eat that at every meal for their whole lives if they want. But the beauty is—they don't. What Satter discovered, and I've found to be true, is that when you provide a variety of options and then back off, it gives kids the freedom to sneak up on foods, try them, and figure out if they like them. I never give my kids

---

* A PDF (http://ellynsatterinstitute.org/cms-assets/documents/203702-180136.dor-2015-2.pdf) summarizing Ellyn Satter's Division of Responsibility may be found at http://ellynsatterinstitute.org/dor/divisionofresponsibilityinfeeding.php.

praise for eating vegetables. I never give them a hairy eyeball for eating nothing but white rice and butter. It's totally up to them.

Now, another part of Satter's philosophy is never to act like a short-order cook. If they don't like what I'm serving, there will always be another opportunity to eat in a couple of hours. Kids get breakfast, lunch, and dinner, plus sit-down snacks midmorning and midafternoon. My kids sometimes whine and say, "But I don't like that! There's nothing at this meal that I like to eat!" To which I reply, "You never have to eat anything you don't like." And the conversation ends there, because they know it's true. I'm not going to force them to eat, not one single bite. After dinner in my house there's never any more food. My kids know that they don't get to graze all day long. They don't get to walk into the kitchen and just open cupboards and start helping themselves.

It might be hard to institute the division of responsibility cleanly if your kids are already older and accustomed to taking what they want from the kitchen whenever they want it. Other than vowing to become an excellent role model and providing good food at mealtime, there may not be much you can do at that point. But if you have young kids and you've been putting pressure on them to eat specific foods, know that you can stop putting all that pressure on them—it will help your children become more competent eaters. Plus it will take a big weight off your shoulders.

What I provide at mealtime to make cooking for a family align with my own Bright Line Eating foods is a big bowl of starch, plus whatever I'm eating—my protein, my vegetable, my salad, my fruit. Good starch options for kids—or any adults in your household who aren't doing Bright Line Eating—include white or brown rice, whole-grain pasta, kamut spirals, quinoa, hash browns, and sweet potatoes. Kids do need some amount of starch. They can't live on just protein and vegetables like we can when we're in the weight-loss phase.

Now, I'm sure that if you're a parent or a grandparent and you've been following along with the science of Bright Line Eating, you've started to get nervous about what your kids or grandkids are eating. I'm nervous about it, too. The options kids are exposed to in restaurants, on kids' menus, and with school lunch programs are horrifying.

I do want to reassure you a little bit. For one thing, it's okay for kids to eat flour. Flour is essentially glucose, and glucose causes problems when it's not utilized immediately for fuel, but little kids use up a lot of fuel. So most of the flour that they eat is getting turned right into glycogen for their muscles and they just burn it right off.

Sugar is trickier. Here's what I do. I don't provide any fruit juice, and I don't provide any soda or desserts. There is no expectation at the end of lunch or dinner that there's going to be any kind of dessert. Not even fruit. If there's fruit, it's served *with* the meal. I don't want my kids to think a wholesome meal needs to be topped off with something sweet.

My kids do use real maple syrup on whole-grain pancakes. They do use honey. But that's about it. There are never cookies, pies, or brownies hanging around. And no chips or really junky, flour-based snacks, either.

When the kids go out to eat, or to a party or a potluck, of course they're confronted with unhealthy options. By and large, my philosophy is not to make a big deal of it. As long as it's not an all-day-every-day thing, research shows that it's not rewiring their brain.[6] What rewires the brain is constant, chronic access. So as long as I'm providing the opposite, I feel like it's the best I can do. I think it's actually worse to heavily demonize those foods, which has been shown to lead to preoccupation with getting them.[7]

My goal is to get my daughters to adulthood acting relatively neutral around food. Of course I'm conscious of trying to minimize the spread of my own food issues on to them. So I'm very careful, for example, *never* to talk about my body or my weight or what I'm eating or not eating around them. I also don't let them talk to me about their bodies in an unhealthy way. I started hearing my daughters mention here or there, at very young ages, that their stomachs were "fat" or a similar derogatory term. I don't even think they knew what they were saying; they were just parroting what kids at school were saying about themselves. I shut that right down. "No thank you," I replied. "No fat talk in our house, please." It stopped happening. Knock on wood.

A final word about the food that other people eat. Many of us are concerned about the eating habits of the other adults in our household, or in our lives. Here is my general principle: Even if there are really solid reasons why I might think a person I love should want to change the way they are eating, I make it a point to not go there. I stay out of other people's food. I "keep my eyes on my own plate." This also means that I need to be responsible for my own food, because if I'm living with someone else who's going to be doing some cooking, it's not my business to make them change the way they cook. It's my business to cook my own food. "I am responsible for the food that I put into my mouth." End of story.

And that includes within the Bright Line Eating community. There are plenty of people who are doing Bright Line Eating successfully and doing it very differently than I do it. Eating things that I wouldn't eat. Eating them in ways that I wouldn't eat them. Or *not* eating things that I *would* eat. Either way, it's none of my business. Honestly, keeping my eyes on my own plate and loving and accepting people no matter what is the only way for me to stay sane.

This is also a great example of how Bright Line Eating helps us in far more ways than just losing excess weight—we develop better boundaries, become less codependent, and separate out eating from social engagement. Don't let your own triumph be undermined by obsessing over someone else's struggles.

Spacing Your Meals

You might be wondering *when* you should eat. The general rule of thumb is to try to eat breakfast at breakfast time, lunch at lunchtime, and dinner at dinner time, and to try to space your meals four to six hours apart. In other words, try not to eat your next meal sooner than four hours after the last meal and try not to wait longer than six hours. I do want to say, though, that this isn't a Bright Line. This is just a guideline. There are times when I eat my next meal sooner than four hours and there are times when I find I have to spread my meals out farther than six hours. Life happens sometimes. But in general, the four-to-six-hour rule is a good guideline.

One of the benefits of waiting at least four hours between meals is that you will have digested your food from the previous meal more thoroughly.[8] If you eat sooner than four hours, you might not have finished digesting the majority of your food, and it's better for the digestive system if you clear out the bulk of the previous meal before adding more.

If you have a tricky schedule, for example you work on a rotating shift, just know that there is always a workable solution for spacing your meals. Here are some of the options people have tried:

- Abandon the "eat meals at standard mealtimes" guideline and go with the four-to-six-hour rule. For example, if you work C-shift, eat breakfast within two hours of awakening, even if that means breakfast in the afternoon, and then space out your meals from there.

- Abandon the four-to-six-hour rule. If your work doesn't give you breaks at regular intervals, you may need to go long stretches between meals, and that's okay. No one ever starved to death between meals.

- Eat two meals a day instead of three. I know some people for whom this is the best solution, because their work schedule is such that they feel they simply can't eat at work, and their life flows much better when they collapse their food intake into just two meals. In general I don't recommend this, but I do know people for whom it works.

- Eat four meals instead of three. Similarly, some people just do better if they can split one of their meals into two, thereby solving, for example, the issue of a workplace that doesn't give them longer than a 10- or 15-minute break at any one time, and they simply don't have time to eat a full meal in one sitting.

You get the idea. The bottom line is, no matter what your circumstances, there's a way to make it work. Remember that the four Bright Lines are *Sugar, Flour, Meals,* and *Quantities.* So long as you're eating discrete meals without grazing or snacking in between, you're doing Bright Line Eating. It's all good.

When You're Sick

If you have a cold, you don't need to feed your cold or starve it, either—just keep sticking to your regular food plan. However, if you've got the flu or a stomach bug and are vomiting, it's a bit of a different story. I do recommend that you still try to keep to a three-meal structure. But you may want to change up the foods you're eating. Try having a breakfast meal for all three meals; foods like oatmeal and bananas might stay down when chicken and salad won't. And, obviously, this is one case when the finishing your food rule goes out the window. If you can only choke down one bite of oatmeal, for goodness sake, stop. Broth is fine if it's weighed and measured at 8 oz. and consumed at mealtime. But the Bright Lines still apply—no ginger ale, no saltine crackers.

A note about colonoscopies. I have never known anyone to be triggered by drinking that stuff so go right ahead and comply with the instructions. If they say you can only ingest clear fluids before the test, take them on a three-meal-a-day structure. Broth or white cranberry juice diluted with equal parts water, plus the prep solution, is fine.

Making Substitutions

The power of Bright Line Eating to bridge the Willpower Gap is that we avoid making decisions about what to eat in the moment based on how we feel. So we never, ever change up our food because we've opened the fridge and thought, "Eh, I don't feel like bell peppers right now. I think I'll have asparagus instead." There's no integrity in that. However, there *are* some legitimate reasons for making substitutions to your food plan.

1. If you've written down fish for lunch and noon comes, you open the fridge, and you discover the fish is rancid, then a) don't eat it, and b) don't drive to the store to buy more fish. Find a different protein, throw it on the scale, and get on with your life.

2. There's something I like to call the "mom exception." Say I've written down roasted chicken, sliced peppers and onions, and salad for dinner. But then my daughter develops an ear infection and I spend the afternoon at the pediatrician's office, followed by a wait at the pharmacy. I arrive home at 6:30 P.M., so there's no way I'm starting to slice onions at that point. It's time to open a can of corn and put frozen veggie burgers in the microwave. Not order a pizza, mind you, just choose more rough-and-ready Bright Line foods. If you don't have kids, you'll probably come across your own version of an unanticipated situation at some point and decide that the sane thing to do is to swap out your precommitted food for a simpler menu. That's fine.

3. Sometimes social factors just make changing your food in the moment the right thing to do. Knowing when and how to activate this option requires some wisdom and perspective, though. These days if the evening comes, we've been cooped up in the house

all day, and my husband says, "Want to go to out for Mexican?" I have no problem saying, "Sure." I've eaten Bright Line meals at Mexican restaurants for years, and making a last-minute swap there feels fine and doable to me. Mind you, I don't do it every day. And in the first couple of years of my journey, I did not make those kinds of last-minute changes. I'd eat what I had committed to, and perhaps plan a dinner out with him for the next day or the weekend, when I could commit to it in advance. It took me a long time to earn back the right to make spontaneous food choices. That said, even in the early days, if I was with girlfriends out on the town and, due to factors outside my control, we ended up stopping at a restaurant, then, yes, I'd eat a lunch out. The most important thing is to not skip meals, or you may open the door for your Saboteur to convince you to eat more food later.

Hunger and Fullness

I want to talk to you about two common bugaboos that have the potential to derail your Bright Line Eating program—and how to make friends with them. The first is hunger, and the second is fullness. I propose that hunger is not an emergency, and neither is being really full. They are just sensations. And you can get used to, and develop a certain level of comfort with, both of them.

A lot of folks start Bright Line Eating having eaten so much so often that it's been a long time since they've actually felt hungry, physiologically speaking. And the only times they realized that they were truly hungry, they immediately went to solve the "problem" by eating something.

Now, in Bright Line Eating, we don't do that. We wait until mealtime to eat. And it's entirely likely and possible that you are going to get hungry before it's time to eat your next meal, especially while you're on the Weight-Loss Food Plan. You're not going to be eating enough food to meet your metabolic needs, which is why you're going to be burning fat stores and losing weight. Under those conditions, hunger is absolutely possible.

It is true that some people go through the Bright Line Eating weight-loss phase and report never feeling hungry. Other people report getting hungry pretty reliably an hour or two before meal-times. And a rare few feel very, very hungry a whole lot. But no matter how you slice it, hunger is not an emergency. It's merely an interesting sensation in the body. But if you don't feel that way, if hunger instills some amount of panic in you, I encourage you to analyze why. Maybe journal about it or learn to make friends with it. It's not excruciatingly painful. It's kind of cute, in a grumbly little way. It's just this little tickle in the tummy. And the neat thing is that usually it goes away. Fifteen minutes or half an hour later, it can be completely gone. Not because you've eaten anything, but just because hunger comes and goes. Often something simple like a glass of water or a cup of herbal tea will help. So I encourage you to start thinking about hunger in a different way. Breathe into it. See what comes up for you when you ask yourself why it frightens you so much.

The twin cousin of hunger is fullness. Now, granted, I'm somebody who actually likes to be really, really full. Before Bright Line Eating, I found something really comforting about that Thanksgiving full-belly feeling, but I have worked with people long enough to know that some feel awful when they're very full. Some folks have reported that the meal size we need to eat in Bright Line Eating is enough to produce that uncomfortable sensation. If you have a history of bulimia and the feeling of being too full is a powerful trigger for you, then cut back the quantities a little bit.

And, once again, I would encourage you to just sit with that uncomfortable feeling and try to make friends with it. Accept it. Journal about it. What is it about the feeling of being full that is scary or uncomfortable to you? What does it bring up for you?

In the past, it's likely that you've reacted to hunger or fullness in a way that didn't ultimately serve your best interests. You now have an opportunity to change that.

Food Thoughts and Mantras

Similarly, you can change how you think about all the "not my food" that's out there in the world. Mantras are a good way to do that. A mantra is any phrase that we codify, imbue with power, and call upon when needed. I have three that have been really helpful to me in my Bright Line Eating journey. The first is, "Don't eat, no matter what. No matter what, just don't eat." Of course, I don't mean become anorexic. I mean don't eat any bite that's not on my food plan. This can be a very comforting repetitive mantra if I'm going through a rough afternoon and driving or walking past temptations. "Don't eat, no matter what. No matter what, just don't eat."

The next mantra that I have found to be really helpful when offered food at parties is, "That is not my food. That's poison to me." I don't say it out loud, just silently to myself. And reframing those foods not as delicious treats, but as deadly poisons, is very effective and very truthful. For me, those foods do poison my life. They poison my body. They warp my mind with cravings and obsessions. They lower my self-esteem. They make me sick. They will make me die decades or years earlier if I continue to eat them the way I did before. They *are* poison to me.

The third mantra is, "Thank you, God, that's not my food." If you don't want any God in there, you could just say, "Thank goodness that's not my food," or just, "That's not my food." In our Online Support Community, this mantra has morphed into a phrase we use often, "Not my food." This is oftentimes abbreviated as NMF. No need to dignify it by spelling it out. It's all just NMF, and you don't have to give it the time of day.

These mantras are part of a more global discussion, which I think is worth having, about our mental fortitude and NMF. I'll tell you a story to illustrate what I mean. I was in Sydney, Australia, six months after I started this way of life, and I had only five pounds left to lose. I was exhausted from severe hypothyroidism that was not being properly treated and the desire to eat had come home to roost. I was battling cravings, valiantly, nearly all day every day. But, up until that point, I was battling them successfully. One day, I was waiting at the bus stop so I could make my way to the University of New South Wales, where I was working as a postdoctoral research fellow. I was standing in front of a café that had cakes in the window—layers of cakes. And, typically, when I stood at that bus stop, I would walk to the next shop, which I think was a bookshop, and stand there so I wouldn't have to stand in front of the cakes.

But I was so exhausted and homesick that day that I allowed myself to stare through the window at those cakes. I didn't just *look* at them, I studied them. I fantasized about how one might taste and how that other might smell and which one I would get if I were going to eat one. In my mind, it was all completely hypothetical. I even said to myself, "I'm safe because I'm not going to eat them. I'm just looking."

I got on the bus and went to work. The next day, I was waiting at that bus stop again. And I walked in and ordered a cake. I didn't stop after one piece—I kept eating. Just like that, I was off on a three-month tear of gaining back all my weight and then some—I went from a size 4 to a size 24 in three months. It was the most painful time of my entire life. I simply could not stop eating.

But, finally, a few months later, I did get back on my program, lost all the weight again, and have stayed slender ever since. What I learned from that experience is that thoughts are very powerful. *I simply cannot afford to let myself fantasize about food.* As soon as I catch myself mentally wandering into the land of NMF, I shut my mind against those thoughts. "That is not my food. That's poison to me. Don't eat, no matter what. No matter what, just don't eat."

Bookending

To end this chapter, I want to talk about a little trick that can help you in any of the sticky situations where you're worried that you might pick up a bite of food that's not on your food plan. This includes going to the movies for the first time since starting Bright Line Eating, grocery shopping at a place with delectables, attending a wedding, or going to a friend's house for dinner. You get the idea. When you know that you'll be facing a tricky situation like that, I encourage you to use a powerful tool called bookending. Bookends go on either side of a row of books on the bookshelf, right? So when you bookend an event, here's what it looks like:

Let's say that the event in question is a wedding. Before the wedding, you could text your buddy or post in the Bright Line Eating Online Support Community: "I'm going to a wedding tonight, and I'm concerned because I haven't ever been to a wedding without eating NMF before. I think it's going to be tempting, but I have my Emergency Action Plan firmly in mind, and I commit to activating it if I get really tempted."

At the end of the event, you come back into the Online Support Community or you text your buddy again and say, "I stuck to my Bright Lines. Feeling awesome! Thank you for your support."

Just knowing in advance that you're going to bookend it, that you're going to report your triumph back to the Bright Line Eating Community or a buddy, will see you through.

Case Study: Meg Queior

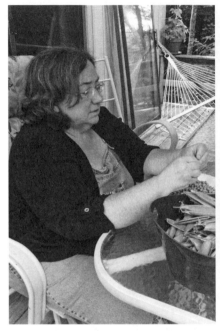 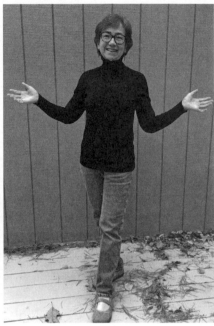

Highest Weight: 261 pounds
Current Weight: 125 pounds
Height: 5'2"

Many of my childhood memories involve food. One of my early memories is of me sneaking into my grandma's pantry to eat clumps of brown sugar out of the bag. Later in childhood, I clearly remember feeling comforted by food and using it to ease my anxiety. By the time I was a teenager, even though only modestly overweight, I was put on diet pills and the grapefruit diet. The need to lose weight was deeply woven into my sense of self.

In my twenties, I'd do things like eat only one yogurt a day. I'd lose 5 or 6 pounds, but it was never sustained—how could it be? Through my thirties and forties, my eating continued to expand.

I tried every diet fad and plan on the market: Weight Watchers (repeatedly), Pritikin, Atkins, the Mediterranean diet, Jenny Craig (as a lifetime member), even a 12-Step group. You name it, I tried it. I would have short-lived, modest success and then regain all the weight, plus more.

By my fifties, my weight had climbed well above 200 pounds. I began taking blood-pressure medication, my mobility was increasingly compromised, and I needed bilateral knee replacements. I felt utterly hopeless about ever finding a way out of my issues with food and weight until a friend connected me to Susan's work. Bright Line Eating helped where nothing else had, not even a 12-Step program for food addiction. The difference for me was that Bright Line Eating explained the brain science behind food addiction. Susan didn't just *tell* me to do something; she explained *why* I should do it. For me, that has made all the difference. Before BLE I called myself a sugar junkie, thinking it was a metaphor, and not realizing that I was hitting the nail on the head.

BLE has been a miracle for me. Within a week, my cravings disappeared. As Susan explained each tool of the program, I picked it up and put it in my pocket. My weight steadily declined. Now my hunger is well-met by my food intake. I enjoy my meals, I'm satisfied, I'm grateful, I move on.

After losing 85 pounds, I happened upon a picture of myself at my heaviest, and it was a revelation. I realized there was some very powerful denial at work that prevented me from fully engaging with my lived reality at the time. It was obvious to everyone else, I'm sure, and in some sense I knew it was a burden, but at my heaviest I didn't actually *see* the weight I carried when I looked in the mirror. To have that reality hit me was quite jarring, and it makes me appreciate the complexity of denial and addiction.

At goal, I weigh half of what I weighed when I started. I am a slow-but-steady loser, so it has taken a while, but that's okay. The journey has been profound. In many ways, it's been easy for me. I don't struggle; I just work the program pretty effortlessly, every day. My well-being has improved across the board: I'm off all medications, my blood work falls in healthy ranges, my blood pressure has gone down, and my newfound mobility is a surprising gift every single day.

Recently I have been thinking a lot about Heavy Meg—who she was and how she felt. It's important to me that I honor her—not reject or deny her. I no longer judge her. I'm learning to be compassionate toward myself, both at the size I was then and at the size I am now. At age 65 and in a right-sized body, life is opening up in rich, deeply satisfying, surprising ways. I have a zest for life that I haven't known in decades, and for the first time in my entire life, I am at peace with my food. I'm convinced that BLE is saving my life. I am deeply, incredibly grateful.

CHAPTER TWELVE

RESTAURANTS, TRAVEL, AND SPECIAL OCCASIONS

Bright Line Living is meant to be resilient and flexible enough that you can do it for the rest of your life, in the real world, with minimal sacrifice. Personally, I am a very social animal. I eat out, I celebrate many holidays with my faith group, and I travel frequently for both work and pleasure. And yet I absolutely stick with my Bright Lines. It's possible to have it all. It does, however, require some extra preparation and planning. In this chapter, we'll be covering living a Bright Life outside your home.

Restaurants

Honestly, I recommend that you avoid eating out for your first 30 days, if you can. It's very helpful to establish the habit of Bright Line Eating before venturing into a restaurant. Eating out is totally possible, but it will always be a bit more difficult to navigate than a meal at home, most notably because you won't be bringing your food scale to restaurants and you'll have to eyeball your quantities. Doing this honestly and without using it as an opportunity to overeat can present an ongoing challenge for some people.

It takes scrupulous honesty not to overeat in a restaurant. If you get a too-large, too-oily meal many times a week, it will keep you fat and ultimately miserable, so it's worth it to learn clean habits in restaurants early on. Don't fudge.

You'll want to choose your restaurants carefully. Go online and look at the menu ahead of time if at all possible. Your goal is to find something to eat in each food category on your food plan. For example, if you're still losing weight and following the Weight-Loss Food Plan, for dinner you need protein, a cooked vegetable, and a salad. If you eat meat, a steakhouse is usually a safe bet because you'll be able to get all three of those things. When you're out to eat, if they don't have any options for one of your categories of food, sometimes you can make some limited substitutions. For example, "produce is produce": you can swap raw for cooked vegetables, or vegetables for fruit. For lunch, if the restaurant doesn't have fresh fruit, you can substitute a salad. However, if you're at goal weight and they don't have a grain that you can eat, you'll have to let it go for that meal.

You will want to order carefully. Let the server know that you don't eat flour or sugar. Order your salad with no croutons, no cheese, and oil and vinegar on the side. If you're not sure what's in something, ask. Request that the food be prepared simply, with no sauces. Make sure fish or chicken is not dipped in flour or breaded.

On occasion, you may have to send your food back. On my twenty-ninth birthday, just a few weeks after I first started following this way of eating, my husband and I were vacationing in New York City. We were in Little Italy in Manhattan, walking around and looking for a nice restaurant. Men with thick accents standing in front of Italian restaurants kept trying to sweet talk us into their establishments. We looked at a lot of menus. I chose a restaurant that had Chilean sea bass, my favorite fish. I ordered very carefully. I told the waiter I didn't eat flour or sugar, and asked him to please grill my fish without dipping it in flour first. The food took forever to come out, we'd been walking all day, and I felt weak and famished by the time it arrived at the table. To my dismay and my husband's incredulity, my fish arrived fully breaded. Normally I would speak up for myself, but in this instance my husband was so blown away by their error that he spoke up. "She said she doesn't eat any flour!" To which the waiter replied, "This is not flour! This is *not flour*! This is *bread*." I always laugh when I think about that night. It wasn't funny at the time though. Now that so many people are following gluten-free lifestyles, that kind of confusion probably doesn't happen often. Take it as a warning to always clearly specify what you can and cannot eat.

When the food arrives, before you start eating, eyeball your portions. Typically the salad and vegetables won't be large enough and the protein serving will be too big. Ask God to help you to see clearly, or invoke your own highest, most honest nature. Then make a cut in the meat so that you have 4 oz. (if you're female) or 6 oz. (if you're male). Take the rest *off your plate* and put it on a side plate. Ask for one if you need to.

In addition to remembering to pray, the trick I use to keep myself honest in restaurants is to imagine myself in a food-weighing contest similar to the "guess how many jelly-beans are in the jar" contests at state fairs. When I'm guessing a quantity in a contest, I'm *really* trying to get it right. I want to win the prize. In a restaurant, I imagine I'm trying to get my estimated weights as accurate as possible so that my "entry" will be the winning one.

In my Boot Camp, I have the time and space to go in-depth on each cuisine, but, in brief, Mexican, Chinese, Thai, Japanese, Indian, and yes, even Italian restaurants are all doable. Here are some tips.

At a taqueria, it's pretty easy to get a burrito bowl instead of a tortilla and then have them add ingredients according to the categories you get in your food plan. Again, estimating quantities is the hardest part, so make it easy on yourself by ordering just one type of protein and then ask for lots of cooked vegetables, salsa, corn, lettuce, etc. Since you'll be combining your 6 oz. of fruit and 6 oz. of vegetables for lunch into 12 oz. of vegetables (or 6 oz. of vegetables and 8 oz. of salad into 14 oz. of vegetables for dinner) you can pretty much ask them to load up the rest of your bowl with whatever kind of produce they have. Then ask for guacamole and/or sour cream for your fat. Voila! If you're at a sit-down Mexican restaurant, fajitas are usually a safe bet—hold the tortillas. Again, stick with one protein source. If you're getting chicken fajitas, leave off the cheese and beans.

At a Chinese or Thai restaurant, you can order vegetables with either meat or tofu, but you'll have to carefully ask for no sugar, flour, or cornstarch in the sauce. I have found that one plate of food in an Asian restaurant is typically the right amount for one meal.

Japanese restaurants can be tricky because they hide sugar in lots of things—the salad dressing is likely to have sugar, but they may not have oil and vinegar available on the side, so you may have to let the salad dressing go. Sushi rice has sugar in it, but if you're on the maintenance plan you can order sashimi and a plain bowl of rice. A side order of edamame makes a great protein serving if you don't like sashimi. A side dish called *ohitashi* is basically boiled spinach; it makes a great vegetable serving if you order it without sauce. If they have a hibachi grill you'll be all set, since a hibachi dinner comes with protein, vegetables, rice (for those in the maintenance phase), and typically some kind of salad (just ask for the dressing on the side). Be careful to state that you don't want them to use teriyaki sauce on the grill, since it's loaded with sugar.

Indian restaurants work well, especially for lunch buffets, but they will be oilier meals than you would cook at home, so you shouldn't eat there often during the weight-loss phase. Avoid the makhani sauce dishes, as they contain sugar. If you're plant-based, you'll find dal (lentils) or chana masala (chickpeas) for your protein, and if you're meat-based they'll have some kind of chicken, goat, lamb, or beef. And there will be vegetable dishes. If you're still in the weight-loss phase, be sure to avoid the vegetable dishes that are loaded with potatoes.

By Italian, I do not mean a pizza place. That won't work, unless they have really bountiful salads. Opt for grilled fish, chicken, or steak with a side of garlic spinach and a salad.

There are two sayings that should become your dining-out mantras: "Less is more," and "When in doubt, leave it out." The goal is to leave the restaurant feeling free, not second-guessing what you ate. If you find yourself thinking about the meal at all after it's over, that's your conscience niggling at you. Journal about it or talk with your Mastermind Group or buddy and figure out what you're going to do differently next time. Create a "next time, I will" contingency plan to help you navigate the situation in the future. For example: "Next time I order fajitas, I will ask for a clean plate and move the sizzling meat and vegetables onto it so I will not be tempted to scrape up every bit of the greasy oil with my spoon."

Travel

If there's one cardinal rule of traveling when you're a Bright Line Eater, it's plan ahead. Plan, plan, plan. There's a great saying about this: If you fail to plan, you plan to fail. It's so true. And the opposite is true, too. With a little forethought, traveling can be really easy and totally lovely. Here are some of the ways that I plan ahead when I'm doing Bright Line Eating.

CALLING AHEAD

If I'm going to be staying in a hotel, I call ahead to find out if I can have a microwave and refrigerator in my room. If not, that's okay, but it affects the foods I'll choose to bring along. If you're going to a conference or traveling with a tour group, call ahead to find out what they're serving for any meals they'll be providing for you. Are the lunches just a sandwich in a box? That's not going to be so helpful. If it's a buffet salad bar with all sorts of veggies and beans, you'll easily be able to make Bright Line choices.

With just a couple of phone calls to caterers and event planners, you can find out if you'll need to bring your own food and how much you'll have to plan for. Oftentimes they'll be happy to provide you with a special meal. Once you've made the call, you can relax.

WHERE TO STAY

If I have control over my accomodations, I prefer to stay in a place where I have access to kitchen facilities. Airbnb has been a game changer for the Bright Line Eating community. Most extended-stay hotels have kitchenettes. Or you could stay with friends or family so that you have access to their kitchen. Hotels work, but having a kitchen is nicer.

BREAKFASTS ON THE ROAD

In general, when I travel I pack my own breakfasts. I just feel like it's easier to start off my day with a meal I don't have to think about—I save that energy for lunch and/or dinner out. I always bring my digital food scale when I travel. I also bring several ingredients preweighed from home. My favorite travel protein is a 2-oz. baggie consisting of mixed nuts, roasted edamame, and roasted chickpeas. (Men would get 3 oz.) For breakfast in a hotel, I'll do one of those baggies, plus 1 oz. of Shredded Wheat'n Bran, and add my own fruit from home, typically an apple because they are easy to transport. If you do have a microwave and refrigerator and you want to bring oatmeal or hardboiled eggs, those are also great options.

PACKING ALL YOUR MEALS

There have been times I have gone to a weekend conference, maybe even a four-day event, and decided that I didn't feel like eating every lunch and dinner in the hotel restaurant. So instead, I've literally packed all my food—veggies, proteins, fruits, and grains, the whole kit and caboodle. It's doable. It's also a good option for people who are really sensitive to oil and salt, perhaps because of a heart condition or GERD. Bringing several days' supply of your own food is an option.

There are two main approaches to doing this. The first is to weigh and measure all of your food before you go and to pack each individual meal into its own Tupperware container. This works best on a road trip, where you can bring a big cooler in your car. When you're at the hotel, you can wheel it down the hall and replenish the ice from the ice machine, then use the drain nozzle to drain it into the bathtub as the ice melts.

When flying, bring your food in the original packaging—not weighed and measured yet—and then bring your digital food scale plus some travel containers. You can weigh it all when you get there.

PACKING NONE OF YOUR MEALS

It's possible not to bring any food when you're traveling, especially if you're a seasoned Bright Line traveler. You might decide to just trust. I've done this plenty and been just fine, but I've traveled a lot—I've taken over a hundred trips since beginning Bright Line Eating. I will go to any length to find a Bright Line meal, and deep down I trust myself to do it. I am not going to cave and eat whatever is being served if it's got sugar and flour in it or if it's not mealtime. I'm just not going to. Even if it's the end of the day and my willpower is shot and everything has gone wrong and the rental car broke down and my suitcase is lost and it's dinnertime and there's a pizza stand right there. I'm not going to go there.

I've built up integrity and trust in myself, but it's taken time. If you're new to Bright Line Eating, I don't recommend going on a trip without a clear idea of where your Bright Line meals are going to come from. It's just not wise. Do what you have to do to protect your precious, precious Bright Line program. It's worth it. Once you've become a seasoned traveler, you might still choose to revert to a more cautious approach to taking trips if you have other stressors going on in your life. I experienced this just recently, after the Bright Line Eating movement started to explode and suddenly I found myself with dozens of employees and thousands of people wanting my time and complicated online technologies to figure out: my willpower was tapped by decision fatigue in a way I had never before experienced. Because of this, I had to stop eating out so much when I traveled. I had to go back to the basics and call ahead, ask what was being served, and go the extra mile to ensure that I would have zero choice-points during my trip. I also had to start taking my scale with me into restaurants—even in my hometown. It may feel weird at first, but I promise you no one is looking. Check my recommended travel scales at http://ble.life/thebook. It's worth it to take the load off that future moment when your willpower might be missing in action. Plan in advance.

FLYING

If I know I'm going to be on an airplane at mealtime, I *always* bring my food. I simply do not trust that I'm going to be able to get a Bright Line meal on an airplane. The TSA will allow you to bring food onto an airplane. What you probably can't do, if you're going through customs, is to take that food *off* the plane. You can't bring fruit or produce into a foreign country.

What the TSA doesn't allow are liquids or gels. So don't pack yogurt, because that's a "gel." Don't bring little containers of salad dressing, either. Just bring it mixed in already.

PLANT-BASED FOODS THAT TRAVEL WELL

Proteins. Little sandwich baggies of nuts, seeds, roasted chickpeas, and roasted edamame (also known as soy nuts) travel well. There are also now vacuum-packed pouches of things like chickpeas in an Indian flavoring sauce—basically just what you would get in an Indian restaurant—by brand Tasty Bite. You just rip it open and heat—it's perfectly good food. It only needs to be refrigerated after it's opened. The pouches can go right in your suitcase.

Grains. If you're on the Maintenance Food Plan, you get grains with lunch and dinner. Seeds of Change makes a quinoa-and-brown-rice mix you just heat in the microwave. If you had to, you could even eat the stuff cold (this is why it's nice to call ahead and find out if you're going to have a microwave in your room). The pouches do not need to be refrigerated, and they're never going to leak, so they're really ideal for travel. Baggies of dry cereal like Shredded Wheat, Uncle Sam's, Ezekiel, or Fiber One are ideal. You could also bring packets of oatmeal.

Vegetables. Veggies are a little trickier because they're often heavy and/or bulky, but packages of baby carrots or sugar snap peas work well. You can also cut up broccoli florets or other vegetables you can eat as finger foods and put them in baggies.

Fats. Half an ounce of nuts or seeds is the easiest fat serving for traveling.

MEAT AND DAIRY PRODUCTS THAT TRAVEL WELL

You might not think of meat and dairy as being foods that travel well, but there are some that really do. The classic example is hard-boiled eggs. They last a very long time, even without refrigeration. You can quickly boil up a dozen, and that's six easy protein servings if you're female or four protein servings if you're male. Just dry them off, put them a baggie, and pack them in your suitcase or bring them in your carry-on. Another really good option is cheese, especially prepackaged string cheeses, which often come in exactly 1-oz. servings. Pack two if you're female, three if you're male, and that's a very convenient protein serving that travels well and lasts a long time without refrigeration. Tuna fish pouches also work well.

FOOD LASTS

When I was first starting Bright Line Eating, I moved to Sydney, Australia. During the two years I lived there, the first and foremost travel lesson that I learned is that food does not go bad nearly as quickly as we've been conditioned to believe it does. I traveled back and forth to the States four times, and went all the way around the world once, and I packed all my meals for those flights. One time, I had a day and half of straight travel time from America back to Sydney thanks to a 13-hour layover in Tokyo, and I ended up sitting down to eat salmon 41 hours after I had cooked and packed it—no ice, no insulated bag, and no refrigeration. It was perfectly fine. Food doesn't go bad as quickly as you think. I'm not adding a disclaimer here; I'll leave you to your common sense.

CROSSING TIME ZONES

The second lesson that I learned traveling from Sydney to America and back is how to space out meals while traveling internationally. At home, standard meal times might be breakfast at seven o'clock, lunch at noon, and dinner at six o'clock. Basically, you're eating every five or six hours. But then you don't eat overnight, which is usually for about 13 hours. So the first time I made the trip, I spaced out my meals as best as I could, doing breakfast, lunch, and dinner four to six hours apart and then leaving a big gap before the next breakfast. It did not go well. I wasn't sleeping for eight hours of that long stretch, so it was incredibly torturous waiting that long to eat.

What I've learned is that when you're traveling, you've got to count all flight time as awake time. Traveling across time zones is grueling. I never set myself up now to be going 8, 10, or 13 hours without a meal if I'm traveling on an airplane.

I've developed a system for figuring out how many meals you should eat if you're traveling across multiple time zones. Now, I'm not talking about traveling across the United States, crossing only three time zones. If you're doing that, it's easy to still just eat three meals a day—a little more spread out in one direction, a little bit more compressed in the other. When you're crossing 6 time zones, or 10, or 16, it becomes particularly necessary to plan out the spacing of your meals, because the notions of "breakfast," "lunch," and "dinner" just don't apply anymore. Night and day are flip-flopping on you.

The first thing to figure out is what your last meal is going to be in the time zone that you're departing. We'll call this an "anchoring meal." For example, suppose you're leaving from home and the flight leaves at 8 P.M. Okay. Then your anchoring meal is dinner. You're going to eat dinner at dinnertime, a couple of hours before your flight. Your next anchoring meal relates to when you land. So let's imagine that you'll be landing at 2 P.M. local time. You want to fuel your body by eating lunch before you land since you'll have to go through customs, find your way to your destination, and get situated in wherever your new place is. You then find yourself dinner at dinnertime in your new local time zone.

So now you've got your anchoring departure meal and your anchoring arrival meal. Count all the hours of travel in between and divide by six. You want to eat every six hours while you're flying. If you have to compress it a little bit and eat every five hours to make it come out evenly, even every four hours, do that, but make sure that you're eating every four to six hours while you're in the air.

BRING YOUR PROGRAM

I just want to remind you of something very important, which is that when you travel you need to plan to bring your *program* as well as at least some of your food. Bright Line Eating is portable, and the last thing you want to do is leave the pieces that give you structure at home and travel to a new location without your tools and the whole system that helps to keep you Happy, Thin, and Free.

For example, my meditation bench is the first thing I put in my suitcase. I also bring my Nightly Checklist sheets, food journal, gratitude journal, Emergency Action Plan, and phone numbers of my buddies and Mastermind Group members.

I have learned the hard way that it is sometimes even more important for me to use my Bright Line Eating tools to stay on plan when I'm traveling than when I'm at home. Traveling is stressful, and there's often a lot packed into a day away—if I don't make sure to take care of myself mentally, emotionally, and spiritually, my willpower will get depleted. I'm going to feel rough instead of relaxed.

So I bring my scale. I bring my support tools. And I continue on with this way of life wherever I am in the world. It goes with me.

Holidays

For many people starting Bright Line Eating, holidays loom large and scary. But let's be real for a minute. Thanksgiving is just a Thursday. You can make it through any given day by sticking to your Bright Lines. You just have to plan ahead and recruit lots of support. Everyone in your Bright Line Community is going to be facing down the same challenge at the same time. We've got you. Eat turkey for your protein, but skip the gravy, and make sure there are some simple, unadulterated vegetables. You can always contribute a dish of your own if you're eating at someone else's house. Mashed or roasted butternut squash is always delicious. Try making a gorgeous garden salad that includes some fresh pineapple, depending on whether it's lunch or dinner. If you're on the Maintenance Food Plan and you get grain with your meal, weigh out some mashed potatoes or wild rice. If you're going to feel awkward bringing your scale to your host's house, treat it like a restaurant meal and eyeball your portions. If you're with family and they know all about your Bright Line Eating program, bring your scale and use it; it will give you peace.

Actually, the traditional Thanksgiving meal lends itself to Bright Line Eating quite nicely. There are almost always foods you can eat. The tricky part is often the timing of the meal. Unless you feel comfortable having lunch (or dinner) at three o'clock, you may want to talk with the host ahead of time and see if it's possible to have the meal at either one o'clock or five o'clock—times that align better with lunch or dinner.

If you're thinking, "No way. I couldn't do this, not on *Thanksgiving*," you are not alone. Many people have that response at first. Listen to this: the first Boot Camp I ever offered started in October, but everyone made it through the holidays and still lost their weight. Research from the National Weight Control Registry shows that people who stick to their food plan on weekends and through the holidays experience less stress and are far less likely to regain their weight.[1] If you want to get thin and stay thin forever, then commit to sticking to your Bright Lines even on special occasions. *It's not going to be as bad as you think.* When you get through your first holiday sticking to your food plan, you'll feel great—but everyone around you will be miserable because they've eaten too much. They'll be moaning and groaning or passed out on the couch, and you'll feel terrific. You may even decide to ditch them and go take a brisk walk, or help with the dishes.

One thing I will warn you, based on my personal experience and that of hundreds of my Boot Campers, is that oftentimes an addictive eater will get through a holiday, vacation, or significant event successfully, but then later, in the privacy of home, end up bingeing as a "reward." It's called "reentry," and it's a real phenomenon. The time *after* a trip, party, or holiday is when you need to keep your guard up and be most vigilant.

Special Occasions

Weddings, birthdays, and other special occasions are much easier to navigate with Bright Line Eating as your guide. You already know what you're going to eat—you're going to eat what's on your food plan. The key is figuring out how to get what you need.

The first rule of thumb is to keep your mealtimes in mind. For example, if the wedding ceremony starts at 7 P.M., you can bet dinner won't be served until after 9 P.M., and that's just too late—you'd be better off eating your dinner before you go. If people ask you why you're not eating, a simple, "Oh, I'm never hungry this late in the evening" will suffice. If it's a 3 P.M. birthday party, don't eat anything there and make sure you get home by dinnertime—but have a packed dinner in your car just in case you end up deciding to stay late.

If the event includes a meal and occurs during your normal mealtime, then by all means plan ahead to eat there. Call whoever's in charge of the food and have a frank and detailed discussion about what's on the menu. If it's a wedding, get the name of the caterer and call them. Caterers typically have no problem making accommodations for guests with special food needs—it's their job. These days everyone is on a special diet—celiacs, paleos, diabetics, etc. Believe me, they're used to it. Just talk through what they're serving and ask for what you need.

When you attend the event, remind yourself to focus on the *people*, not the *food*. Play this little game: See if you can meet three new people, remember their names, and learn two interesting facts about each of them. Test yourself on the way home. You'll be surprised how much the added human connection will enhance your enjoyment of the evening.

I also encourage you to focus on what you'll enjoy about the event now that you've begun your Bright Line Eating journey. Is it wearing a dress you haven't fit into for a long time? Dancing without feeling self-conscious? Feeling more confident meeting new people? So many members of our community say that what they love now about holidays and special occasions is that they really feel like they have something to celebrate—their new life.

Case Study: Nathan Denkin

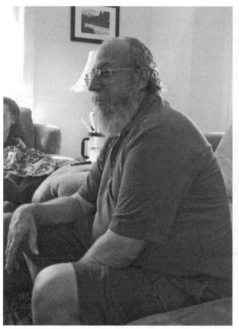 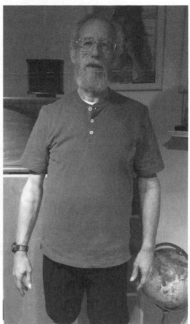

Highest Weight: 235 pounds
Current Weight: 155 pounds
Height: 6'0"

I'm one of those people who grew up naturally thin and, while that may seem enviable, the downside was that bad habits crept in and took hold, then eventually caught up with me. By the time I realized that I weighed 235 pounds, I had decades of poor food choices under my belt—literally. Pizza, ice cream, double-bacon cheeseburgers, I loved them all. When I was diagnosed with Crohn's disease, the prescribed corticosteroids accelerated my weight gain. Deteriorating discs and related spinal problems caused me to drop my calorie-burning activities.

At age 66, I was diagnosed with coronary artery disease. I was certainly motivated by that. I got down to 183 six months later, but then six months after that I was back up over 200. I truly felt stupid, although I had always considered myself to be a pretty intelligent person. I skipped a grade in elementary school and was in honors classes in high school and college; I have a Ph.D. from Caltech in physics and I worked at Bell Labs. But when it came to food choices, I acted like an imbecile. I realized I had done damage to my body that I was going to have to live with forever.

Then, at 67, I found Bright Line Eating. In many ways, the biggest blessing was finally learning why I had previously failed to keep the weight off. It may not sound like much, but when you can't accept the bad choices you were making about food for so long, knowing the reason for those choices is important. Before Bright Line Eating, even getting to 180 seemed like a stretch goal. Being able to finally set a goal weight according to where I needed to be for optimum health was amazing. Actually reaching it? There are no words. With the weight off, my triglycerides dropped 36 percent. My blood pressure dropped so much that I had to get off the metoprolol that I was taking for atrial fibrillation. I reduced my dose of aspirin as a blood thinner from 325 milligrams to 81 milligrams. My doctors often have more questions now about how Bright Line Eating works than about my health! Best of all, my energy level is greatly improved and I sleep better.

As a scientist myself, what changed my life the most was getting answers to questions I didn't even realize I had. Perhaps for the first time in my life, I understood myself and why I'd made the choices I had, even when they worked against my own self-interest.

Happy, Thin, and Free applies to far more than my weight and food issues. This program shows me how to apply what I've learned in all my endeavors to live a happier and healthier life.

CHAPTER THIRTEEN

WHAT IF I BREAK MY BRIGHT LINES?

You might assume that it's not a question of *if*, but *when*. However, I know many people who have gone 30 or even 40 years without ever crossing their Bright Lines. Once you establish Bright Line Eating as a lifestyle, there is *absolutely no need* for you to break your Bright Lines. Ever. One day at a time.

This is a point I really want to emphasize, because people often fail to realize how truly possible it is to stick to their Food Plan for years, without deviating. Not because you're fanatical, just because *it works*. Do you remember the discussion in Chapter Seven about how ingrained habits don't drain our mental energy, like brushing your teeth twice a day for years on end? It's the same.

In fact, I want to expand upon this analogy a bit, because I think it's illustrative. Many of us brush our teeth twice a day, every day. And, while I'm sure we all believe it's a worthwhile behavior, we probably don't think of it as being the foundation of our happiness, health, and sanity. We also don't imagine that some great tragedy would transpire if we skipped brushing occasionally. Yet we stick with it, faithfully, morning and night, day after day because a) we believe we're better off brushing our teeth than not, and b) once the habit is established, it's easy to stick with.

The benefits of Bright Line Eating go way beyond decent breath and healthy gums. For many, adhering to the basic habits of this program triggers a cascade of powerful transformations. Stubborn weight that clung for decades melts off; the need for medications vaporizes; energy soars; chronic health problems disappear; self-confidence grows; hearts burst with quiet bliss. Private jigs are danced in department-store dressing rooms. Closets get organized. Dawn is greeted with wide and grateful eyes.

Behind this, for many, runs a fear—a niggling uncertainty or, worse, a paralyzing panic—that one deviation from the Bright Line Eating Food Plan would send the whole structure crumbling to rubble, and land us right back at square one. This fear, valid or not, rational or not, is the magnetic force that repels our fork away from any bite of food that's not on the plan. We know that no momentary satisfaction can be worth it.

The habits of Bright Line Eating become as ingrained as the habit of toothbrushing, so we get most of our steadiness for free. It's easy. Early morning flight? No worries, the baggies of travel foods are already preweighed from the night before and ready to toss into the knapsack. Wedding on Friday? Better call the caterer today and line up our meal. Road trip? Fun! Cooler's packed. Bright Line meals at rest-stop picnic tables four to six hours apart get woven into the itinerary.

So, the combination of automaticity, extreme elation at the health-joy inherent in our new lives, and horror at the thought of returning to our old existence keeps us on the beam.

That said, I am well aware, after over 20 years in various different 12-Step food programs and having coached thousands and thousands of people through the Bright Line Eating Boot Camp, that many, many people will break their Bright Lines at some time or another. And the points I want to make about that are: a) it's not worth it, so if you haven't done it yet, don't; b) look at a lapse as a strengthening experience, not a catastrophe; and c) remember that you can always, *always* get your Bright Lines back, though it will be easy for some and hard for others.

I have not been perfect about sticking with my Bright Lines since I started this way of life. I've traveled a rocky road and done a lot of research on what works and doesn't work for my brain. I can share my personal experiences about the range of what can happen when you break the Bright Lines. Before I do, though, I want to remind you that I'm a 10 on the Susceptibility Scale, which means that the consequences for me are more dire than they would be for someone who's a 4. In fact, the lower you are on the Susceptibility Scale, the less likely it is that you'll choose to aim for strict adherence to the Bright Lines under every condition anyway.

After the incident with the cake in Australia, followed by my painful and dramatic weight regain, I eventually got my Hashimoto's disease—a type of hypothyroidism—and extreme adrenal fatigue under control and started my weight-loss journey again. Once my brain healed the second time, I had a more typical Bright Line experience—my energy returned in full force and I had very few cravings. As the weight came off I felt increasingly exuberant, and after that, I followed my food plan precisely, with no breaks for about two years.

And then, on December 5, 2005, while in a yoga class, I was watching the teacher do a demonstration when I suddenly blacked out with no warning and fell straight back, like an oak tree.* Once in the ER, I was floating in and out of consciousness for quite a long time, coming to and asking, "What happened? Where am I?" and my mom would explain, and then I'd be in a coma again for a while, and then I'd come to and ask again, "What happened? Where am I?" My brain was swelling up.

In the midst of this, apparently, I told the doctors and the orderlies and the attendants, "I'm a recovering drug addict. Please don't give me any drugs." According to my mother and husband, I was quite emphatic. I said it over and over. "You can't give me any drugs. I'm a recovering addict."

---

* I had recently given up all condiments and, more significantly, all salt, in an attempt to get as simple and pure as possible with my food. Low blood pressure runs in my family, and, unbeknownst to me, my blood pressure was running about 75/50. I also have a condition called neurocardiogenic syncope, which means I am prone to fainting. The solution is simple, and has been prescribed by doctor after doctor after doctor. I must salt my food. Heavily. Lesson learned.

Of course, when I finally regained normal consciousness I was in excruciating pain. I said to the first person I saw, "I am in *so much pain*!!! Why haven't you given me anything for this?" And they said, "Well, you told us not to." And I replied, "That's ridiculous. I change my mind!" So they did end up giving me something to kill that pain. Thank goodness.

When I got out of the hospital, I did the strangest thing. I went straight to the grocery store and bought binge food. Lots and lots of binge food. My husband was livid. He had been through the wringer with me and my food addiction, seen me gain all my weight, lose all my weight, gain all my weight back in Australia, and finally lose all my weight again. At that point, I had successfully abstained from sugar and flour for two years, so the idea that I would throw all that away and go back to bingeing on ice cream and pies was horrific to him. When he asked me what I thought I was doing, I replied stubbornly, "I'm hungry. I need to eat. I'm going to eat. Leave me alone." Not only did I buy ice cream and pies, but I bought cigarettes. And for the next two-and-a-half weeks, I just binged and smoked cigarettes. Nonstop. It was awful.

Then I went to my follow-up appointment with the neuro-surgeon. His first question was: "Are you having any issues with impulse control?"

I started to sob.

It turned out that when my head hit the hardwood floor at that velocity, not only did I fracture the base of my skull, my brain slammed back and then ricocheted forward. On the rebound, it hit the front of my skull, which is cragged inside, like a coral reef. The frontal lobes got bruised very badly from the impact. They were swollen, immobilized, and essentially not functioning.

He said, "Your prefrontal cortex is the seat of impulse control, judgment, and decision-making, and it's useless to you right now. The swelling will take about two more weeks to go down, but when it does, you'll find that all the circuitry you've developed in your years of building good habits will still be there. You'll be fine. But right now, you can't access that part of your brain at all." I knew what the prefrontal cortex was, of course, and all this made perfect sense to me. It was a huge relief.

Sure enough, two weeks to the day after that doctor's appointment, I stopped eating addictively. It was like a light switch turned back on. I went back to weighing and measuring my food and sticking to my Bright Lines. It was easy.

It's noteworthy to me that I didn't pick up any drugs or alcohol during that period of time. At that point, I had been clean and sober for over 11 years and my identity, on the deepest level, had become that of someone who does not ever, under any circumstances, use drugs or alcohol. Even when large parts of my brain were taken offline, another part of it worked to protect my recovery.

By contrast, I'd "only" been off sugar and flour for a little over two years. My deepest identity had not yet become cemented as someone who does not eat sugar or flour under any circumstances. It's interesting how long it can take for a wholesale shift in identity to happen.

It's also interesting that, toward the end of those awful days of bingeing and smoking, it dawned on me, at some point, that I couldn't even taste the food. *At all.* The scientist in me got curious, so I went to the store, got some supplies, and did some blindfolded taste tests. Chocolate vs. vanilla ice cream? Nope, couldn't taste the difference. Brie vs. peanut butter? Nope. They tasted the same.

Apparently, I had lost my sense of taste in the accident.

Did that keep me from bingeing?

Not one bit.

On and on and on I ate, and the fact that I couldn't taste the food was irrelevant. That's when I really internalized the fact that we don't overeat because of palatability or mouth feel, or because we love it—we overeat to scratch an itch in our brains. We might as well be injecting a needle full of sugar and flour into our arms.

The neurosurgeon confirmed that I had lost my sense of smell in the accident, and with it almost all of my sense of taste. I asked if I would ever get it back. He said he couldn't be sure. The neurons running between my nose and my brain had severed straight through; if the break was low in the neuronal pathway, the nerves would grow back, but if it was higher up, they wouldn't. He said my odds were 50/50.

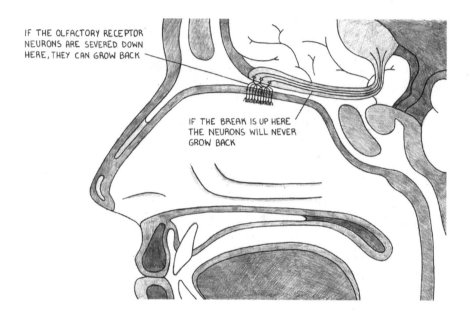

IF THE OLFACTORY RECEPTOR NEURONS ARE SEVERED DOWN HERE, THEY CAN GROW BACK

IF THE BREAK IS UP HERE THE NEURONS WILL NEVER GROW BACK

I'm happy to report that, over the next several years, my senses of smell and taste gradually returned. I'll never be a food critic though, and don't ask me if a room smells funny. I have only the vaguest idea.

For the next six years, I stuck to my Bright Lines without an exception. Not a single baby carrot at three in the afternoon, not a bite, lick, or taste off-plan. And what's interesting to me about that time is that some of the most painful and intense experiences of my life happened during those six years. It started when I was diagnosed with infertility and we went through rounds and rounds of fertility treatments. Eventually, we got pregnant—with twins. They were due August 16. But I went into labor on April 25. Alexis and Zoe were born a week later, weighing under 1½ pounds each. They spent nearly four months in the neonatal intensive care unit. Zoe came close to death many times. There was a 4 percent chance that they would both survive and be healthy. It feels like a miracle that we made those 4 percent odds and they are both doing fabulously well today, but it was a harrowing time in our lives to say the least—and I didn't eat off my food plan.

The birth of our third daughter, Maya, was nearly as horrific. For me, not her. She was born at full term, by C-section, but my spinal block completely wore off during the surgery. Meaning five hours of feeling *everything*. And it got worse from there. Three weeks of a spinal headache worse than any migraine—it's caused when the hole at the spinal block insertion site doesn't close and all your cerebrospinal fluid leaks out, leaving your brain rattling around in your skull. Bleeding ulcers from the pain meds left me vomiting up blood every day. And I had two three-year-olds running around, needing me, and a newborn keeping me up all night.

I *still* didn't eat off my plan. Not once. There were times when, due to the ulcers, my Bright Line meal consisted of only 4 oz. of white rice and 8 oz. of whole milk to coat my stomach, but I weighed it precisely, even while doubled over in pain. That's all I ate—not one bite more.

How?

I had built up a strong foundation. I had the proverbial "reserves in the bank." Automaticity was in full effect, and my brain just did what it knew how to do. Write down food the night before. Commit to it. Eat only and exactly that. Wash. Rinse. Repeat.

So yes, it is possible to stick with the Bright Lines for years and years, *no matter what* life dishes up.

Breaking Our Bright Lines

To help you understand the Bright Line philosophy about breaking the lines, I need to give you some background context on the programs I attended that formed the kernel of Bright Line Eating.

As I've mentioned, the first 12-Step program for food that I tried didn't take an explicit stance on sugar, flour, or other addictive foods. We met to talk about our compulsive overeating and to support each other in our individual efforts *not* to overeat, but everyone functioned autonomously in defining what that meant for them. There were no Bright Lines. In meetings, we would talk openly about the excess food we'd eaten, how we'd deviated from our plan, and what new plan we were going to try next. That was part of the culture. I experienced a lot of mutual tenderness, camaraderie, and spiritual growth—but no actual physical recovery. This was true for most of the other participants as well. I left that program just about as sick or sicker with food than I had been before I joined. And certainly way, way heavier. That was eight years of my life.

I eventually found a different 12-Step program, which dealt specifically with *food addiction*. It gave a ton of specific guidance on weighing and measuring food and rules about not eating sugar or flour. These were clear: As soon as you broke them, you were restricted from speaking at a meeting for 90 days. You couldn't do service work. You had to stop sponsoring others, and you were kicked out of your 12-Step working group.

That severity served to silence the narrative around discussing openly, in the community setting, what it's like to break the Bright Lines and then come back. I watched people who struggled to go long stretches without a deviation get closer and closer to the shadows and feel more and more marginalized because they didn't have a voice. And I imagine that it felt isolating, shaming, and ostracizing.

In Bright Line Eating, we create an environment that includes the best of both worlds. We celebrate the strength in our shared commitment to sticking with the Bright Lines. A commitment to no exceptions, to being unstoppable. This gives us the physical recovery we're seeking—lasting weight loss and brilliant health—and it also results in a lot of freedom and happiness. This is what's so counterintuitive for people who don't need Bright Line Eating. Having a clear structure can lead to so much freedom.

However, we also understand and celebrate the lessons we learn from moments of imperfection and we welcome that narrative and that experience into our community. If you break your abstinence, we don't isolate you. Instead, we have a dedicated Support Community to help you get back on track. Others have been through the same thing, and they can help you find the lesson in your experience. We find that there's a lot of strength and insight, wisdom and healing that emerges when we remove all judgment from the community and foster only love, acceptance, and a fierce commitment to ongoing growth.

The Four S's

Think of all the yo-yo dieting that goes on. All the people who lose a huge amount of weight and then turn around and gain it right back.

There's a lesson there: *the most important part of any attempt is how you respond when you miss the mark.*

There is a huge difference between a successful, helpful, adaptive response to a break and an unsuccessful, unhelpful, maladaptive response. It's the difference between living the rest of your life Happy, Thin, and Free and retreating into the shadows to eat in shame, with another failure logged in your personal loss column.

There are four key components to handling a break in our Bright Lines successfully, adaptively, and in a way that strengthens us. They are the Four S's.

1. SPEED

The first is how quickly we can do what we call in Bright Line Eating, not resuming, but "rezooming." You don't want to fall prey to the "what-the-hell" effect. This is a technical term in the psychology of eating literature[1] for the mental phenomenon that happens in chronic dieters when they have broken their diet. It's not uncommon to think, "Well, I might as well eat everything under the sun since I broke my diet anyway. I'll start over on Monday." Or, "I've had one bite of pizza; I might as well eat the whole pizza and a half gallon of ice cream while I'm at it. I'll start my diet again later."

No. Let's go get back on track. Like, now. Not tomorrow morning. Not Monday, not on January 1. Now.

Speed.

To be fair, I know that not every moment is right for rezooming. Sometimes we're just in the grip of our food addiction and we're simply not willing—or able—to stop eating. And that's okay. But even in those moments, we can watch, in a detached and calculated way, for an opening that will allow us to hop back onto our Bright Line path. We can pray for willingness. And we can implement the other three S's. They will help us get back to the other side.

2. SELF-COMPASSION

Can we be loving with our inner self-talk? Instead of beating ourselves in self-flagellation, can we try nurturing ourselves the way we would a friend who has called us in crisis? Use the same tone with yourself that you'd use with a best friend who just sprained her ankle on a hike. You'd get her help. Rally resources. Make sure she was resting and taking it easy. An example of a helpful thought is, "I just ate a bunch of sugar, so I know my thinking is going to be really negative and irrational for a day or two, maybe three. My head is going to try to get me to feel desperate about everything." No spiral. Shame over eating leads to overeating.

Just be gentle, kind, and encouraging. You are not a bad person. You just have a malfunctioning brain.

3. SOCIAL SUPPORT

In my experience, the first thing that comes up after a break is a profound desire to *isolate* yourself. This manifests as not wanting to reach out to anyone. You just want to hide, eat, and deal with it alone. But that is not a good idea. Shame flourishes in silence. The most effective thing to do when you've had a break is to reach out to other people who do Bright Line Eating and who are walking this journey with you. Let them know what happened and how you feel. Let them help you construct your plan to get back on track. They can probably see what you need much better than you can at that moment.

You might need a buddy or a Mastermind Group. I needed to commit my food each day, to a human being, live on the phone, for a long time. If you haven't gotten enough social support so far, you might want to revisit the section on buddies and Mastermind Groups in Chapter Ten and start to build a posse.

If the breaks keep coming and there seems to be no end in sight, if you're a 10 on the Susceptibility Scale and are feeling totally powerless, that's a sign that you need to try something different and radical. Consider hiring a Bright Line Eating coach. Examine what you've been doing so far, reread this book, and figure out how you're going to up your game. You've got this.

4. SEEK THE LESSON

My friend Pat Reynolds says, "Every break can be turned into a breakthrough." And he's right. There is almost always a powerful lesson to be found in breaking the Bright Lines. If we envelop ourselves in shame and isolation, we'll probably miss the opportunity to learn from the lapse. After every break you should absolutely take an inventory of your life, mental state, thinking, and behavior leading up to the first bite. Odds are, you're not fully using the tools available to you. Are you overly busy? Not letting yourself rest? Putting off meditation? Not using your Nightly Checklist Sheet? Or is it something else, like you can't stand to say no to other people's food offerings in social situations? Whatever it is, it's a growth opportunity.

The Permission to Be Human Action Plan

The Permission to Be Human Action Plan is a ten-question process that will help you find the lesson and growth opportunity after you've broken your Bright Lines. It will also have a positive, calming effect on the negative thinking that can crop up after a break. The ten questions are included in the back of this book in the Resources section. I think you'll find this to be a very powerful recommitment process, and I encourage you to keep it with your Emergency Action Plan, or somewhere you'll always have it handy, even if that means writing it down and folding it up in your wallet. I want you to be able to access it at a party or other social situation. Excuse yourself to use the bathroom, and take yourself through these questions mentally. But I also recommend, when you can, getting somewhere private so you can *write out* your answers to those ten questions. Answering them longhand will make all the difference. You may even want to post your answers in the Online Support Community. I'm sure other people would get a lot out of your experience, and we would love to support you in your recommitment journey.

I want to end this chapter by saying that there's a continuum of sticking with the Bright Lines. There's sticking with the Bright Lines perfectly from Day 1, which I relate to, celebrate, and honor. The moment I stopped drinking and using drugs, I committed to adhering to those Bright Lines. And then, on the other end of that continuum, there's struggle and barely being able to string two days together of Bright Line Eating. I relate to that, too. In Sydney, Australia, when I went from a size 4 to a size 24 in three months, I was doing everything in my power to stop eating and *I just couldn't*, until the tsunami of food addiction receded. It took what it took. Both are different experiences of traveling the same path.

Most of us, most of the time, experience something in the middle. Regardless, Bright Line Eating is a community for everyone. That whole continuum of experience is welcomed here and is honored here, and there are lessons to be learned at all points of that continuum. Typically, people who are struggling feel like everyone else is more successful and no one else breaks their Bright Lines or is pinned down by the food the way they are. And people who have never had a break feel like everyone else is breaking and rezooming and they wonder if they're all alone in their steadfastness. But in Bright Line Eating none of us are alone. The reality is that every possible permutation of Bright Line Eating is being experienced fully, every day, by hundreds—if not thousands—of people.

But if you are doing Bright Line Eating and it's going well, *protect that.* Your Saboteur, I guarantee, will try to convince you to try an exception here or there. *Don't fall for it.* That road is slippery and painful. The knowledge that rezooming is possible should *absolutely not* be used as an excuse to take a slight detour from the Bright Lines and then try to get back on track right afterward. It doesn't work like that. The first thing that happens when you break the Bright Lines is that your freedom evaporates, instantly. And it goes downhill from there. You don't want to live a life full of the drama and anguish of breaking and rezooming. The reason we honor the Bright Lines and commit to living within them is because we find that consistency and structure make us Happy, Thin, and Free. More than that, they allow us to be the people that we strive to be and to do more of the things we want to do in life. Our focus moves beyond food; we become self-actualized and engaged with the world. *That* is what we all want our lives to be about.

That said, if you're reading this section because you've broken your Bright Lines, never fear. I want you to know that you can come back from that, and that living Happy, Thin, and Free is still on offer for you. Because in Bright Line Eating, we are not called to be *perfect*. We are called to be *unstoppable*.

Case Study: Colleen Egan

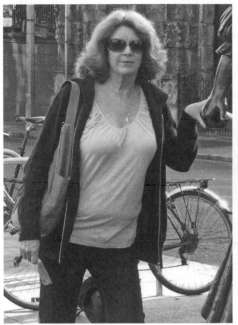 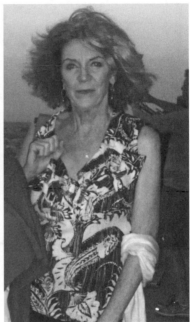

Highest Weight: 197 pounds
Current Weight: 142 pounds
Height: 5'9"

At age five, I climbed up on a countertop to reach into the cupboard for a box of brown sugar. While I was in elementary school, my uncle worked for Frito-Lay and he would bring over cartons of chips when he visited. I wanted to eat them all, but settled for eating as much as I could before they were taken away from me. Then, later, I would sneak back to eat some more.

I was 11 when I realized eating was a problem for me. I ate more than anyone else and always wanted to keep eating when everyone else was done. I was taller than my mom, my older sisters, my brother, and my girlfriends. I was called the Jolly Green Giant by a boy in the neighborhood, and that label stuck for many years. In high school, we all wanted to be like Twiggy. We tried not to eat so we could all be just as thin. That didn't work! But, since Twiggy was so revered in the media, she became the model to emulate. I internalized that I was huge, and a failure.

As I got older, I started hiding my eating, all the while bingeing on sugar and flour. I also think that the commercial introduction of frozen convenience foods and fast foods during my youth had a huge impact on me. Easy grab-and-go. No preparation needed, just put it in the oven—and later, the microwave. If one is not enough, it's easy to make another. They're small, after all. I remember when it became unpopular to cook. The media only showed the benefits of processed foods.

As I aged, I invested more and more energy into trying to lose weight. I bought multiple books and magazines, and would follow their plans to some short-lived effect. I tried quick-loss schemes like the cabbage soup diet. I even tried eating *only* ice cream, cookies, and cake to try and make myself develop an aversion to them—it didn't work. I started serving meals on smaller plates. I tried putting my fork down between bites and chewing my food for a ridiculously long time. I tried to drink a liter of water before dinner. I ate only one meal a day. I ate an apple one hour before dinner. I switched to low-fat processed foods. I ate only packaged foods so I could accurately measure my calories—yuck! I read labels and tried to avoid things with high sugar content and hydrogenated oils. I started using olive oil, the "healthy" oil. I listened to people who I thought had the answers and tried to follow their advice. I tried to eat healthfully. I went on vacation with one of my sisters, who controls her weight, but when I tried to mimic her eating pattern I found it just wasn't enough food for me.

I desperately tried to find the balance. Nothing ever worked. I got more and more frustrated, angry, and disillusioned. Then, a few years ago, just after the New Year, I decided I could not make any more weight-loss goals. I could not "diet" anymore. I gave away my collection of over 30 diet and nutrition books! I would not go back to Weight Watchers or Jenny Craig. I just could not face any more deprivation, rebound weight gain, or failure. I resolved to accept myself as I was; I just didn't believe I was capable of controlling my eating.

At the same time, I knew I had to improve my overall health. I had high cholesterol and prediabetes. It was a time of great conflict for me. My doctor said if I didn't lose weight she'd just have to keep increasing my medications until I finally wound up on insulin; but *I couldn't* lose weight. After 40 years of dieting, I was still more than 30 pounds overweight. I decided to try to learn how to cook vegetables, via an online cooking class with Katie Mae, in the hope that increasing my vegetable intake would help . . . somehow.

That vegan cooking class was the turning point. Several weeks in, Susan Peirce Thompson showed up as a surprise guest speaker. *Serendipity*! I felt understood, finally! The science she presented made sense. I knew I was high on the Susceptibility Scale.

I took one more chance with altering my diet, and it worked. I'm still working it!

When I started Bright Line Eating my A1C was down to 5.2 from 5.6, but I was taking metformin. At that time, I was also taking simvastatin and had total cholesterol of 307 with triglycerides 126, LDL 216.

I stopped the metformin when I started Bright Line Eating. Six months later, after having lost 30 pounds, my A1C was 4.9! I also stopped taking simvastatin when I started Bright Line Eating. Six months later, my total cholesterol was 205 and one year later it's 193, with triglycerides down at 73 and LDL at 113. My HDL remained unchanged, and averages 65 to 66.

I love how I feel. I love not having to struggle with clothes. I feel a level of confidence that I never had before. I'm enjoying the variety and quantity of foods that I eat. I'm able to entertain, dine out, and travel while maintaining my Bright Lines!

Best of all, I'm more calm and accepting now. I'm more gentle and honest with myself, and with others. I'm not as driven to "get it right," which has improved all my relationships. I truly feel like I got a second chance at life.

Part V

GOAL WEIGHT, MAINTENANCE, AND BEYOND

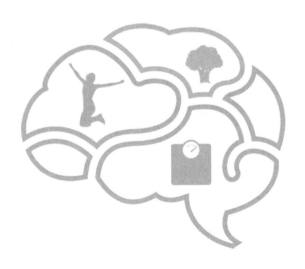

CHAPTER FOURTEEN

GETTING TO GOAL WEIGHT

You might be surprised to find a whole chapter devoted to this topic. You might be thinking, *I'll just do the Weight-Loss Food Plan until I'm thin and then I'll switch to the Maintenance Plan—easy*! But actually, it's a little more complex than that. This chapter is all about ensuring a smooth transition from one to the other. We don't want you to fall short of your goal—or blow right past it and have people start to ask if you have cancer. This has happened frequently enough that I now make sure to spell out how to slow your weight loss. To start, we'll talk about how to figure out your goal weight.

Goal Weight

Right off the bat, I will mention that your goal weight is likely going to be much lower than you think it is. Now, don't misunderstand—I'm not here to force you to get skinnier than you feel comfortable being, or to say that skinnier is better. It's just that, over and over, I have found that people's idea of what's possible for them, or maximally healthy for them, has been skewed by years of being overweight and trying and failing to change. Understandably, they're cautious about setting a bold, unbiased goal. They've lost sight of what a right-sized body really is for them. And that's okay.

The point is that Bright Line Eating restores choice in the matter. *You choose* your goal weight. Personally, I've found a point at which my body disappears—in my mind's eye. I hardly think about it. When I sit down, I don't wonder whether rolls are visible from the side. When I get dressed, I consider the color and cut and style—or comfort—of my clothing instead of worrying about whether it conceals bulges and bunches.

If you've ever been in a right-sized body as an adult, even if you have to think back to high school or college, the weight you were at then is probably your goal weight. I don't care if you're 70 years old now. You'll get there. Go ahead and laugh. I've seen it happen too many times to have any doubts.

If you've never been in a right-sized body as an adult, you can try using a formula to get a general sense of what to aim for.[1] Or not. Oftentimes my Boot Campers will just set an initial goal weight, knowing full well they may reevaluate as they get closer. I think that's a perfectly reasonable strategy. Sometimes setting the true goal weight at first just freaks people out. I worked with a woman recently who is 5'2" and has never been under 200 pounds as an adult. The idea that her goal weight might be between 110 and 115 pounds was just too weird for her to sit with. Odds are, she'll get there, but initially she's setting 140 as her goal weight. And that's fine. What seems impossible right now might seem effortlessly within reach six months from now.

So once you've zeroed in on your goal, how do you get down there? Over the years of working with people, I've come to think of it like landing a plane. You've been cruising at altitude on the Weight-Loss Food Plan for quite a while, and now you need to make some careful calculations to arrive at your destination. You can't keep circling the airfield indefinitely. Some things need to change to land this plane. And you want it to be a soft landing. I'm going to be the flight controller who helps you coast right down to the runway and live at your dream destination forever.

Plateaus in Weight Loss

Certain individuals (with low basal metabolic rates) can experience plateaus in their weight loss. But don't freak out if your weight hasn't changed for a week—a plateau means not losing any weight for more than four weeks straight, with *immaculate* Bright Lines. If it happens, less food is required. For starters, avoid nuts, starchy veggies, and fatty proteins. If, after two weeks, weight loss hasn't kicked in, make the following modifications in sequence, spaced two weeks apart. First, replace both breakfast and lunch fruit with 6 oz. steamed greens. If needed, then reduce lunch and dinner fats to 1 teaspoon. If needed, then reduce all proteins to ¾ serving (female) or ⅔ serving (male). Keep your Bright Lines bright. At the commencement of maintenance, the foods may be restored in the reverse order they were removed until a stable goal weight is achieved.

Slowing Your Weight Loss

If your weight loss is humming along, then, at some point, you'll need to transition to maintenance. The general idea is to *gradually* add more food to your plan until your weight loss tapers off and you are exactly at the weight you want to be.

It's a process.

First, once you are ten pounds from your goal weight, you need to start weighing yourself at least weekly. Monthly weighing isn't frequent enough to give you the data you need. Daily is fine, too, but, for this transition process, it's the weekly numbers you want to focus on.

The key factor for determining your next steps is to figure out, on average, how fast you are losing weight. The options are: Super-Fast, Fast, Medium, and Slow. Super-Fast is 2.5 to 3 pounds (or more) per week. Men are way more likely to fall into that category. Fast is 2 pounds per week, on average. Medium is 1.5 pounds a week, and Slow is 1 pound (or less) per week.

If your weight loss has slowed down over time, use your current rate of weight loss. Once you have determined your category, you're ready to read on. As you're thinking about this, remember, as I explained in Chapter Eight, it's a myth that it's not healthy to lose weight fast. Nor should you despair if you are slower to lose. We're all on the same Happy, Thin, and Free journey, and, for all of us, the maintenance phase of the trip is the longest part, by far. In each and every case, the weight-loss phase is precious and relatively short. Some just transition sooner than others. It's not necessarily a blessing. Each trajectory has benefits.

To glide gently into maintenance, add food in the order suggested below. Keep in mind that if you are averse to certain foods (like grains), you can substitute by adding servings of other foods (like vegetables, fats, or proteins) instead.

Here are the steps for adding food as you transition to maintenance:	
1.	Add 4 oz. cooked grain to lunch
2.	Increase breakfast grain to 1½ servings
3.	Increase breakfast protein to 2 servings
4.	Add 4 oz. cooked grain to dinner
5.	Add 1 fruit to dinner
6.	Increase lunch grain to 6 oz.
7.	Increase dinner grain to 6 oz.
8.	Increase breakfast grain to 2 servings
9.	Increase lunch vegetables to 8 oz.
10.	Increase dinner fat to 2 servings
11.	Increase lunch fat to 2 servings
12.	Increase lunch grain to 8 oz.
13.	Increase dinner grain to 8 oz.
14.	Add 1 oz. nuts to breakfast
15.	Add 1 oz. nuts to lunch
16.	Add 1 oz. nuts to dinner

A TYPICA
FEMALE
MAINTEN
← FOOD PL
INCLUDE
ADDITIO
1–4.

A TYPICA
MALE
MAINTEN
← FOOD PL
INCLUDE
ADDITIO

SOME
ATHLETE
ESPECIA
← ACTIVE
INDIVIDU
EAT THIS
OR MORE

Adding Back Food

Here's what to expect, based on the experiences of thousands of people:

1. Changing your Food Plan may scare you. You have been so committed for so long to eating a certain way that adding food may feel like you're doing something wrong. It might be super uncomfortable. You may feel resistance to going through with it. But at this transition point, adding in food means making a *healthy* choice for yourself. So lean in to the Online Support Community or your Mastermind Group and breathe through it.

2. You're likely to be terrified of gaining your weight back. This is also a completely natural response to changing things up after months of watching the weight pour off your body. As long as you continue to stick to your Bright Lines, that won't happen. *You won't regain your lost weight.*

3. Your weight may indeed pop up right away when you add back food. THIS IS NORMAL. Keep that food in, and continue to be precise with your weighing and measuring. Within a week or two, if not sooner, your weight should come right back down to where it was. Then, after your body has stabilized with the additional food, you should start to lose weight again. That's when you add in the next element. Keep watching. If, a week later, you're still losing weight, add more food. If not, wait and watch. It's a process.

SLOW WEIGHT LOSS

You have it the easiest. Stay on the Weight-Loss Food Plan until you are at your goal weight. Then add one element of food. The table says the first thing to add is 4 oz. of grain at lunch, but if you're typically hungrier before lunch than you are before dinner, you may choose to increase your breakfast first. In which case add #2 and then #3 first to get your breakfast up to your Maintenance level. Remember to keep in mind what I said above—your weight may pop up a bit. It's temporary. Just hold steady.

Some people do live forever on the Weight-Loss Food Plan because it just happens to equate to the right amount of food for their body. But if you've been losing weight and you're getting down to goal weight, that's probably not you. You're probably going to need to add at least a little something to stabilize.

MEDIUM WEIGHT LOSS

Add your first food element—either to lunch or breakfast (see above)—when you're within 2–3 pounds of your goal weight. Then follow the directions for Slow. When you have added enough elements to stop losing weight, you've found your Maintenance Plan.

FAST AND SUPER-FAST WEIGHT LOSS

If your weight loss is Fast, add your first food element when you're five pounds from goal weight. If it's Super-Fast, add your first food when you're ten pounds from goal weight. Then follow above.

The Dance of Maintenance

Note that for many, if not most people, goal weight can fluctuate a bit, and living at maintenance is like a dance. Odds are you're not going to settle on one food plan and stick with it forever. Bodies change, metabolisms change, notions of what "goal weight" should be change, and you will probably need to add or take away food accordingly. Weighing yourself at least weekly during maintenance is recommended. You'll want and need that data to inform your journey.

How You'll Look

You may, as you get down to goal weight, look gaunt, especially around the face and neck. This often reverses after a few months at goal weight, even without gaining any weight back. Fast weight loss just seems to work that way. So set your family's expectations. Reassure them that you're not doing anything unhealthy and your rosy cheeks will return.

Similarly, brace yourself for many of your friends, family, and acquaintances expressing concern about your weight loss. Expect them to make comments like, "You're not going to *lose any more*, are you?" They may say this when you still have 20 (or even 50!) pounds to go. Smile, thank them for their concern, and share about it in the Online Support Community. Somehow, the eyes of our society have gotten broken and, since it's a cultural anomaly for people to go from being heavy to truly slender, it undoes people. Don't take on their freak-out. You're fine. Bring it here, to your Bright Line Eating buddies. We get you. And, after you've been at goal weight for a long time, people will relax. They just want to make sure you're not anorexic or aiming for 70 pounds.

Skin

First, I must reassure you that not everyone winds up with loose skin. We have Bright Lifers who have lost over a hundred pounds, and their skin rebounded. Others have had loose skin, waited about a year to see what would happen, and then have decided to have it surgically removed. This isn't always covered by insurance, but sometimes it is. One woman, Sharon, got it covered because she was developing sores where the excess skin was rubbing and her doctor successfully appealed on her behalf. Some also walk a path of acceptance. As we say, "Thank goodness for clothes."

Which leads to the conversation about whether we'll actually be happy with our bodies at goal weight. In general, it's an emphatic "Yes!" People tend to *love* what they look like after Bright

Line Eating. But, let's be real: most bodies do not conform to the ideal pushed on us by airbrushed magazines and photoshopped ads. We may have loose skin; we may have had children; we may simply be older. In my view, we need to develop and maintain a certain humility about our bodies as we age. We'll probably never look like bikini models, and that's okay. Our bodies are so much more than their appearance. And, accordingly, what Bright Line Eaters seem to revel in most of all is their rediscovered agility and vitality. Activities that they had been barred from for years are now in play again. And lives that felt like they were foreshortening are opening up. *And*, I have watched literally thousands of people become radiant with joy at their appearance. Both are true.

Do I Have to Do This Forever?

Not that long after I gave birth to my third daughter, my older two were emerging from toddlerhood and reaching an age where I really started to have misgivings about weighing and measuring my food in front of them. I've taught psychology of eating classes—I'm familiar with the research that shows how mothers' neuroses about food get passed on to their daughters very easily.

In my course, in the unit on feeding children, I taught Ellyn Satter's "Principles of Competent Eating."[2] As I mentioned in Chapter Eleven, she believes that, so long as you maintain the structure of only eating at mealtimes, you should give yourself permission to eat, with focus and respectful attention, whatever you want in whatever quantities you want. *Permission* is the key to competent eating, and anything else qualifies as crazy neurotic.

At that point I had been working the 12 Steps for 18 years. I could safely say there were no unexamined issues left, no harbored emotions to eat over. My pond felt like there were no ripples in it. I remember saying the words, "I can't even *imagine* hurting myself with food these days. Why would I do that? I just wouldn't anymore."

So I decided to make a change. I took it very seriously. I set up support for myself. I got a coach and I made a list in my smartphone of 20 or 30 people who would support me in the endeavor. And with that, after six years of immaculate adherence to my food plan, I ate a brownie. I ate it mindfully. I took deep breaths. I savored every bite. It was delicious. I didn't want another one. I chalked it up as a win and walked out into the world to be a competent eater.

What I found was that suddenly, managing my food felt like a job again, and the job got more and more burdensome. My weight started to climb a little bit, which I expected, but I didn't want it to climb any higher. So now I was back in the game of having to control it. The mental game of: *Am I going to make an exception tonight? Am I going to eat less lunch because I'm going to have a bigger dinner? I need to make sure I exercise in the morning because I had more food yesterday. If I leave work and have cake and ice cream at lunch, because that's what I really want, will I be able to stop there? Or will permission turn one serving into five?* It just became insane. And the insanity started to spiral wider. I had three little kids and a full-time job, and, frankly, I didn't have time for it. My life rapidly became unmanageable. Pretty quickly, I realized competent eating wouldn't work for me if I wasn't willing to get heavy again, which I simply wasn't. So I tried other things. I was doing "research" after all, so while I was at it I tried every other approach I could think of to manage my eating and my weight. But my standards were very, very high. I knew I wanted to be *Happy, Thin,* and *Free.* I would settle for nothing less. But nothing worked. I could never recapture the freedom I had enjoyed for so long. And I most definitely was *not* being a better role model around food for my daughters. After about eleven weeks of very conscious, dedicated effort, I waved the white flag and gave myself the gift of following the Bright Lines again.

What was going on in my brain during all of that? Given that the Bright Lines had allowed me to feel like I was living in the world as a 2 or a 3 on the Susceptibility Scale for many long years, why was I not able to continue being neutral around food when I abandoned the Bright Lines? Why did my Susceptibility Score immediately start to creep back up to 10, even though I wasn't eating to avoid inner issues, or eating to numb myself from the "burdens" of life?

The neurology here is that our daily behaviors form actual physical "rivers" in our brain called fiber tracts. Even if we later divert the neural energy in a new direction and form new fiber tracts, what we leave behind is like a dry riverbed. It never goes away. Our new habits divert the water to flow somewhere else, but it's possible for that water to revert back to its old course again. And that's what I found. The dry riverbed of my old food addiction was just there, waiting for me.

I've said this before—but the point might hit home more poignantly now—this is the reason the Susceptibility Scale Quiz asks you to think back to the time in your life when your eating was at its worst. That's when you formed your deepest riverbeds. You might have grown a lot, and your eating habits might be much better now, but you're still physically susceptible to using those old channels. Your brain still sees them as eligible pathways.

It's worth restating that my brain had gone very far down the path of addiction. There might be other people who have not had as intense an experience, and they probably rank as 3s or 5s on the Susceptibility Scale. So, despite everything I've said here, you might decide to do your own experiment. One of my favorite sayings is that I never deny anyone their "research." God knows I have had to do mine.

Essentially, you've got two choices: stick with the plan and enjoy your new life, or try the experiment of deviating from it to see what happens for yourself. In my experience, most people find that the benefits of living Happy, Thin, and Free go away very quickly when they stop doing the things on a daily basis that got them Happy, Thin, and Free in the first place.

Sooo . . . if you want to *live* Happy, Thin, and Free, and not just subject yourself to another temporary weight-loss success followed by demoralizing subsequent weight regain, you might just find, like me, that once you get to goal weight you do indeed need to stay true to the daily habits that made it all hum and purr from the start. By then, that might actually sound like a pretty good deal.

Case Study: Sharon M.

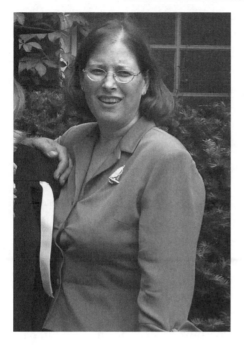 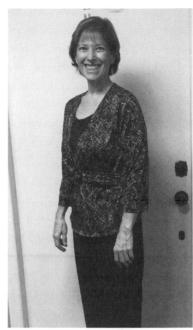

Highest Weight: 165 pounds
Current Weight: 110 pounds
Height: 5'3"

Ever since I was a child, I've suffered from being overweight. There are a few photographs of me as a happy child, but what I remember most is the sadness and isolation. My father was an alcoholic, my mother was trapped in a situation she couldn't contend with, and we children were caught in the middle. Food became a comfort . . . a friend . . . something to turn to when there was no one to talk to. My father also had real issues around sugar, so candy and sweets were a normal part of my young life. My earliest recollection of a binge was taking a box of frozen doughnuts from the freezer, hiding, and eating a few before I realized there was no way I could conceal the "evidence" of what I'd done. I was ashamed, but couldn't stop eating—even at eight years old.

My weight continued to rise as I grew; kids, adults, and even teachers treated me differently because of it. No one "saw" me or gave me the attention a child needs for comfort or guidance. So, food remained my solace, my go-to when I was angry, tired, bored, or sad. Hunger was not the cue for my eating. In fact, I seldom felt hungry, but I ate constantly because I had so much anxiety. As a teen I made the diet rounds: Weight Watchers, Atkins, and pills—all before my sixteenth birthday. I had some success, but the issues of how to navigate the loneliness and how to *maintain* the weight loss were never addressed.

As I got older, I was able to use exercise and regular dieting as a way to control my weight. But at 5'3" and a high of 165 pounds, I felt unattractive, masculine, and aging. I also had thinning hair. Many more diets followed: Overeaters Anonymous, CalorieKing, Dr. McDougall's, and Whole Foods Plant-Based. I even consulted a nutritionist with a Ph.D. and went on vitamins, shakes, and detoxing regimes. It drove me crazy. Why was I so driven to eat sugar and refined food? Why would I send my husband out for a food run at 7 P.M. when I was too tired to go myself? Why couldn't I solve this mystery? I'm intelligent, I have degrees in nursing and business management, I'm certified in nutritional counseling, and I teach yoga. Why couldn't I conquer this issue?

Then, one summer, I took care of my grandchildren for a week. After eating a "kid-friendly" menu for so many days, I felt miserable. Flying home, I went into a sugar stupor. Then my husband and I stopped at a fast-food restaurant for dinner before getting home to an empty refrigerator.

That evening, tired from the trip and loaded up on refined food, I felt desperate. I prayed to God to help me and that very same evening, in an e-mail, a friend shared the Bright Line Eating "Friends and Family" video with me and celebrated her recent success. I immediately Googled Bright Line Eating and read everything I could find online. I realized it mirrored a 12-Step food program, so I started the next day. No sugar, no flour, three meals a day, and measured quantities.

Within just a few days, I started to sleep better and feel better. By the time the October Boot Camp started, I had already lost 20 pounds and questioned whether I even needed to sign up. But my BLE friend kept reassuring me that this was so much more than just a diet—that this program had the tools to help me achieve meaningful and long-lasting change. And wasn't that what I really needed? Not just another diet, but tools for life, and perhaps even the dream of weight maintenance?

My weight loss was not fast, but it held steady at an average of 4.5 pounds a month. I weigh 110 pounds now and feel totally comfortable with the maintenance program and my goal weight range. I have committed to be on the Bright Line Eating plan for the remainder of my life, one day at a time. I no longer eat sugar or flour and actually don't really desire or want it. This program is enough for me.

My hair is healthier, my skin is clearer, and my nails are stronger. I feel giddy when I see myself in size 4 or 6 clothing, and now I can even wear a belt! I know my brain is healing because my long-standing anger and depression issues are lifting. I've had melancholy and anxiety my whole life, so I just assumed I was wired that way. Now my mood is even and high, and I feel real joy each day. I sleep six or seven hours a night and awake rested most mornings. My long-standing hip and toe pain is mostly gone. My yoga practice is deeper, as my muscles have lengthened even more. My energy level is getting better all the time.

I have embraced this program with two strong arms. I don't question it—I just follow it. It has been my lifeline, and I know that it is the answer for me. One day at a time!

CHAPTER FIFTEEN

CONCLUSION: LIVING HAPPY, THIN, AND FREE

The best thing, in my experience, about living Happy, Thin, and Free is that it's not so much a state of *body* as a state of *mind*. I find that many of my Boot Campers report feeling Happy, Thin, and Free long before they reach goal weight. This powerful new state of mind occurs because a distinct transformation happens in the brain when we do Bright Line Eating, and in this last chapter I want to give you a sense of that magic.

Happy

We scientists are just starting to learn the scope of how eating well affects the brain. But you won't need science to tell you: you'll feel it. You'll simply start to feel happier. Better. Brighter. Bounce-out-of-bed good. The doldrums will lift and you'll have a sense that life is finally working for you.

In fact, many people find that they no longer need antidepressants or other forms of psychiatric medication after they've been doing Bright Line Eating for a while. Of course, work with your doctor(s); nothing in this book should be taken as medical advice. Some people absolutely need to stay on their medication.

But, in my experience, many—perhaps a majority—end up weaning off successfully.

Why does this happen? There are at least four reasons.

The first is that eating little to no processed foods leads to a better mood. Sugar, in particular, is a known depressant.[1]

The second is that eating lots of fruits and vegetables is correlated with high mood and low levels of anxiety and depression. In studies, teenagers who ate vegetables for a day reported feeling happy immediately afterward.[2] Adults who eat vegetables every day have less depression and anxiety than those who eat them less frequently,[3] and increasing the number of servings of fruits and vegetables makes them correspondingly happier.[4]

Third, achieving the right balance of omega-3 to omega-6 fatty acids in our diet increases happiness and lowers depression. Your brain is about 60 percent fat, and these essential fatty acids are the most critical molecules for determining its ability to function, perform, and heal.[5] Critically, omega-6s should outweigh omega-3s at a ratio no higher than 5-to-1, but ideally 2-to-1, or even 1-to-1.[6] Omega-6 has become incredibly prevalent in the Standard American Diet because soybean oil—and other vegetable oils—have crept into everything. Packaged foods like crackers, cookies, chips, salad dressings, and mayonnaise are pumping us with omega-6 fatty acids at levels that are beyond our capacity to manage. These days, most people's ratio of omega-6 to omega-3 is an appalling 15-to-1 or even 25-to-1.[7] But when we stop eating packaged foods, voila! We lower our omega-6 consumption dramatically, and that brings our ratio into balance, which leads to enhanced mood. If you want to facilitate this process, eat things like wild salmon, chia seeds, and flax seeds, which are loaded with omega-3s. But just eliminating all sugar and flour will do the bulk of the work for you.

Last, the good food that we're consuming in Bright Line Eating, like blueberries, kale, and fruits and vegetables in general, not to mention chewing our food rather than simply gulping down soft calories, increases a precious and super-important process called *neurogenesis*—the formation of new neurons in the brain—which research shows increases serotonin and improves mood.[8]

Thin

The most important thing I have to say about getting thin, which might surprise you, given how much I sing the praises of losing weight, is that I think being *thin* without being *happy* and *free* is totally useless. I know that so, so many of us just want to get thin. But "thin" doesn't necessarily mean "well," as there are many ways to get thin—like taking methamphetamines or getting sick—that are not what we want at all. Thin, however, does feel amazing when it's done the right way and when it's paired with *happy* and *free*. When your slender body is earned, and you watch yourself nurture and love yourself with the food you put in your mouth each and every day, it feels really, really good.

One of the reasons Bright Line Eating works so well to keep you thin for life is that it sets a bar, and then the bar doesn't move. The expected behaviors are clearly defined, and they don't change. There's no fooling yourself about whether you're doing them or not. Once you've lived a Bright Line life for even a few days, you have a formula that you know works. After you reach your goal weight, if a couple of pounds creep back on, you can take a quick inventory, see where you're off track, and make the necessary adjustments.

For me, after so many years of pouring all my effort into losing weight and never getting anywhere close to goal, suddenly being thin and staying thin felt like a fairy godmother had waved a magic wand and turned me into Cinderella on the night of the ball. It was pure heaven. And, in many ways, it still is. There are so many good things about being thin. Clothes not only fit, they look good. Even jeans! Even swimsuits! I no longer have to stash perfectly good clothes in the back of the closet because I've outgrown them. Now I wear my favorites for years until they *wear out*. I love going to the pool with my kids and feeling confident. I love getting dressed up for special occasions, putting on something formfitting, and knowing that I look lovely. I love being able to touch my toes and tie my shoes without strain or help. I love being able to roll around on the floor with my kids and hug my knees up to my chest. I love that, when I make the time to lift weights, the results show right away because there are no layers of fat hiding my muscles. I love feeling like my outsides match how I feel on the inside. I love showing up in a right-sized body to greet the world. Or going to a job interview or event and not worrying about what I look like or whether I'll be judged negatively because of my size. I love standing next to my husband, meeting his friends and colleagues, and not worrying that my appearance reflects poorly on him. And I love *not having to think about losing weight* so I'm freed up to do what I'm meant to do in this world. And that brings us to . . .

Free

Sometimes someone who ranks super low on the Susceptibility Scale will ask me, "What does the 'free' mean?" When that happens, I momentarily want to trade brains with them. It means *freedom from food obsession.* Freedom from thinking about your weight. Freedom from having a running conversation in your head about what you ate, what that means about what kind of person you are, what you're going to eat, what that will mean about what kind of person you are—that exhausting, endless loop of food shame and food plans.

We cannot underestimate how much space the conversation about our weight has been taking up in our brains. It is *literally* a waste of our lives. I have so many wonderful, challenging things to think about and focus on, from my work to my marriage to my friends to my kids. I know you do, too. I don't want to spend another second of my life using my brain space to make trades, make deals, make plans, and run the numbers, run the numbers, run the numbers. Whether those numbers are pounds, calories, or miles, it's a toxic conversation. It ends here.

Another huge benefit of adopting the habits of Bright Line Eating is that you'll become more resistant to willpower depletion. Your initial willpower won't get stronger, but *your brain* will get stronger at functioning even when confronted with all the things that deplete it. And what's awesome about that is that your new-found strength will spill over into all kinds of other areas of your life. You'll do your laundry more often, quit smoking, find that you don't want or need caffeine anymore, that you don't procrastinate as much, and that your closets are suddenly clean. Research bears this out,[9] and I see it again and again in the Boot Camps.

With your excess weight gone, your life in order, and your other pesky bad habits falling away, you'll step into a new reality. Lighter. Freer. You'll have time on your hands, space in your brain, and amazing new avenues of purpose and meaning will open up for you. You'll be the best version of yourself, able to pursue the most cherished and long-ago-abandoned longings of your heart. And *that*, my friend, is the purpose of Bright Line Eating—to unleash the human potential that's trapped underneath the excess weight that plagues two billion people on this planet.

The Future of Sustainable Weight Loss

The goal of Bright Line Eating is to become known as, and to be scientifically proven to be, the most effective weight-loss program in the world. But that requires long-term data. We are now tracking our graduates and can't wait to see where they are 10 years and 20 years out.

The data we have now are based on relatively small, self-selected samples, because we only have information from people who have filled out our online surveys. Hence, the numbers I'm about to present can't be extrapolated to the population at large. That said, what we're already witnessing is different, in dramatic ways, from the typical results of other programs. A study covering Weight Watchers[10] and another study using prepared meals supplied (for free) by Jenny Craig[11] showed that after *two years* on their programs, people had net losses of about 8 or 9 percent of their starting weights. For example, a subject who started at 160 pounds would lose 14 pounds total over two years.

In contrast, during a typical *two-month* Bright Line Eating Boot Camp, survey respondents have lost, on average, 10 percent of their starting weight, or 19 pounds. That's *more* weight, *12* times faster. And this average *includes* those who join the Boot Camp to manage an eating disorder and *gain* weight.

After the Boot Camp ends, 87 percent of respondents maintain their weight loss or continue to lose weight. Within one year, 28 percent are at goal weight, and many more are still losing. At goal weight, on average, the group has lost about 25 percent of their starting weights. So, for someone who starts at 160 pounds, they lose, on average, 40 pounds. Many, of course, lose much more.

Of those at goal weight, so far, 84 percent are maintaining it. Eighty-four percent! I'd love to tell you how much higher that is than other programs, but I can't, because there is NO OTHER EATING PROGRAM ON THE PLANET that has a cohort of people reaching an ideal weight and then maintaining it.

Here's what our research shows: The people who are successful are those who are committed to keeping sugar and flour out of their system. The people who use all the tools of Bright Line Eating stay on track.

As I have said before, I am not the Bright Line Eating police. I will not come to your house to check whether you're writing down your food or using your Nightly Checklist Sheet. But the data are clear. Those who commit to doing the program as it is laid out heal their brains and move on in right-sized bodies like no other group of dieters.

The Future of Weight-Loss Research

I am super excited that Bright Line Eating works, and that thousands are experiencing the profound transformation that has meant so much to me in my life. But we've just begun. And the big, broad vision is to dramatically, I mean *dramatically*, change the future of obesity, weight loss, nutrition, and health, the world over. To move the dial. Push the envelope. Change the narrative. Forever.

By 2040, I want to see *one million people* living at goal weight with Bright Line Eating. That's our Everest Goal.

And, scientist that I am, here's what I know. It's going to take *research.*

We've got to prove that Bright Line Eating works over decades, study the factors that are most crucial for its success, advocate for insurance in the United States (including Medicare and Medicaid) to cover the Boot Camp so the poorest and hardest-hit can have full access to *all* the tools, and incorporate new technological innovations as they become available.

We're already doing research at Bright Line Eating and partnering with academics and other groups. And the nonprofit research foundation I cofounded, the Institute for Sustainable Weight Loss, is looking to collaborate with scientists around the world to answer the next phase of questions, including those below.

Long-Term Weight Loss and Associated Health Outcomes

How many people are able to stick to Bright Line Eating over the long term? How many people stay at goal weight indefinitely? What is the impact on their psychiatric medication prescriptions, blood pressure, heart disease, and diabetes?

Neurobiology of Addiction

How long does it take for the dopamine receptors in the nucleus accumbens to replenish after people stop eating sugar and flour? Why does bread scratch the itch in some brains, while candy does the trick for others? Why are peanut butter and bacon common binge foods if they don't contain sugar or flour? How does the Susceptibility Scale play into all of this? Do the brains of thin people who are high on the Susceptibility Scale look like the brains of obese people?

Nutrition and Weight Loss

How do fat and animal protein affect health and weight loss? Right now, most people who eat a lot of animal protein also eat sugar and flour—as do most vegans. I'd like to look at omnivore versus vegan Bright Lifers over the long term and see if, when sugar and flour are taken out of the equation and the diet includes lots of vegetables, small amounts of meat, dairy, and fat have less of a health impact.

Joy

I never could have imagined, when I lumbered around UC Berkeley with marshmallows in my pocket, that I would ever be someone who feels good in a bikini. That I would spend all of my thirties feeling energetic and unencumbered by my body, and move into my forties feeling the same way. Happy. Productive and on track. I am so grateful that I discovered a way of eating that catapulted me into this new dimension of living. And that I was able to piece together the science to explain to myself and to thousands of others *why*.

Honestly, the emergence and growth of this Bright Line Eating movement feels like a miracle to me. A miracle as big, or bigger, than the personal weight-loss transformation I experienced myself well over a decade ago, which started this whole thing. As I write this final section of the book, in the dark, past midnight, in the passenger seat of a Ford F-150 pickup truck as my husband drives and our three little kids sleep in back on a road trip across the United States, I am flabbergasted. Thanks to the power of the Internet, in a relatively short period of time, with just an e-mail list, a weekly blog, and a simple two-month online course, thousands of people, from over 75 countries around the world, have collectively lost over 300,000 pounds. And just over a year ago, those numbers were 50 countries and 100,000 pounds. We are mushrooming incredibly rapidly. At every moment of the day, we are online supporting each other, loving each other, and feeling connected.

Every dimension of joy, celebration, and freedom is being shared among us.

And I have no doubt: the best is yet to come.

Wherever you are today reading this, however long into the future, however you feel in your heart right now, however tired you are of the struggle and the disappointment, I want to leave you with *hope.*

You are not alone. There is a way out. There is a road map, and *it works.*

I'm going to end by asking you to visualize yourself in the not-too-distant future, having committed to Bright Line Eating and having lost all your excess weight.

For real.

Close your eyes and go there.

Imagine waking up in the morning, grateful to be alive and feeling simply *wonderful.* Your two feet hit the floor and you stretch. Your arms fall down along your sides and your elbows tuck in, feeling the narrowness of your torso. There's no pain in any of your joints. You bend over. Your hands touch your toes and you bounce there for a while, feeling light and nimble.

You're confident. You know you're aging as well as you possibly can and taking great care of your health. Your mood is high and stable.

You walk over to your closet. All the clothes are the same size, and they all fit. Every last item. You know that when you get dressed you'll feel and look great. You're a walking billboard. People often ask, "How are you so joyful?"

Every day is just like this. You feel excited to greet the world and bask in the pride of friends and family. You have found a host of new friends on this Bright Line Eating journey, and your world is expansive and endlessly enriched. You're excited about the new projects you've started, your new direction in life. There are no barriers. You are the person you always knew you could be.

This is you. Feeling unstoppable.

This is you. Happy, Thin, and Free.

It's not just a tagline. It's a way of life.

RESOURCES

Sample Nightly Checklist Sheet

At http://ble.life/thebook you can download a version of the Nightly Checklist Sheet that you can then modify yourself. While you're visiting our website, be sure to check to see if we've been developing any amazing new digital tools for you to use!

Nightly Checklist Sheet

MON: _____	TUES: _____	WED: _____	THURS: _____
☐ I committed my food for the day.	☐ I committed my food for the day.	☐ I committed my food for the day.	☐ I committed my food for the day.
☐ I asked for strength to have a Bright Line Day.	☐ I asked for strength to have a Bright Line Day.	☐ I asked for strength to have a Bright Line Day.	☐ I asked for strength to have a Bright Line Day.
☐ I weighed myself just once. _____ Change _____	☐ I weighed myself just once. _____ Change _____	☐ I weighed myself just once. _____ Change _____	☐ I weighed myself just once. _____ Change _____
☐ I made my bed.	☐ I made my bed.	☐ I made my bed.	☐ I made my bed.
☐ I read something spiritual or uplifting.	☐ I read something spiritual or uplifting.	☐ I read something spiritual or uplifting.	☐ I read something spiritual or uplifting.
☐ I meditated for _____ minutes.	☐ I meditated for _____ minutes.	☐ I meditated for _____ minutes.	☐ I meditated for _____ minutes.
☐ I wrote down what I will be eating tomorrow in my food journal.	☐ I wrote down what I will be eating tomorrow in my food journal.	☐ I wrote down what I will be eating tomorrow in my food journal.	☐ I wrote down what I will be eating tomorrow in my food journal.
☐ I wrote in my gratitude journal.	☐ I wrote in my gratitude journal.	☐ I wrote in my gratitude journal.	☐ I wrote in my gratitude journal.
☐ I wrote in my Five-Year Journal.	☐ I wrote in my Five-Year Journal.	☐ I wrote in my Five-Year Journal.	☐ I wrote in my Five-Year Journal.
☐ I am getting to bed in time to get 7–8 hours of sleep.	☐ I am getting to bed in time to get 7–8 hours of sleep.	☐ I am getting to bed in time to get 7–8 hours of sleep.	☐ I am getting to bed in time to get 7–8 hours of sleep.
☐ I stuck to my Bright Lines today! Day _____	☐ I stuck to my Bright Lines today! Day _____	☐ I stuck to my Bright Lines today! Day _____	☐ I stuck to my Bright Lines today! Day _____

FRI: _____	SAT: _____	SUN: _____
☐ I committed my food for the day.	☐ I committed my food for the day.	☐ I committed my food for the day.
☐ I asked for strength to have a Bright Line Day.	☐ I asked for strength to have a Bright Line Day.	☐ I asked for strength to have a Bright Line Day.
☐ I weighed myself just once. _____ Change _____	☐ I weighed myself just once. _____ Change _____	☐ I weighed myself just once. _____ Change _____
☐ I made my bed.	☐ I made my bed.	☐ I made my bed.
☐ I read something spiritual or uplifting.	☐ I read something spiritual or uplifting.	☐ I read something spiritual or uplifting.
☐ I meditated for _____ minutes.	☐ I meditated for _____ minutes.	☐ I meditated for _____ minutes.
☐ I wrote down what I will be eating tomorrow in my food journal.	☐ I wrote down what I will be eating tomorrow in my food journal.	☐ I wrote down what I will be eating tomorrow in my food journal.
☐ I wrote in my gratitude journal.	☐ I wrote in my gratitude journal.	☐ I wrote in my gratitude journal.
☐ I wrote in my Five-Year Journal.	☐ I wrote in my Five-Year Journal.	☐ I wrote in my Five-Year Journal.
☐ I am getting to bed in time to get 7–8 hours of sleep.	☐ I am getting to bed in time to get 7–8 hours of sleep.	☐ I am getting to bed in time to get 7–8 hours of sleep.
☐ I stuck to my Bright Lines today! Day _____	☐ I stuck to my Bright Lines today! Day _____	☐ I stuck to my Bright Lines today! Day _____

Permission to Be Human Action Plan

Learning to live HAPPY, THIN, AND FREE is a process. There is no perfect straight line to success. It's a journey, and every journey has steep uphills, gentle downhills, and nice stretches of flat land. There are gorgeous vistas and horrible storms. You'll get blisters. You'll see sunrises. You'll go until you don't think you can take one more step . . . and then you'll go some more. Pretty soon you'll be a seasoned trekker.

One thing that can derail us is thinking that we must be perfect.

There is no perfect.

But there is progress.

This "Permission to Be Human Action Plan" is offered with love as a road map to follow in the event that you find yourself on the other side of the Bright Lines, and you want to get back on track.

Ask yourself these questions:

1. What was the situation? What happened?

2. What led up to it? How had I been feeling?

3. What sabotaging thoughts did I have right before I picked up the bite?

4. How do I feel now that I've crossed the Bright Lines?

5. Did I write down my food last night?

6. Have I been using my Nightly Checklist Sheet and other tools?

7. Did I take any actions to protect my Bright lines before eating?

8. What could I do differently next time?

9. What have I learned?

10. What action can I commit to taking RIGHT NOW that will support me in my Bright Line Eating journey?

ENDNOTES

Preface

1. Ng, M., Fleming, T., Robinson, M., Thomson, B., Graetz, N., Margono, C., . . . Gakidou, E. (2014). Global, regional, and national prevalence of overweight and obesity in children and adults during 1980–2013: A systematic analysis for the global burden of disease study 2013. *The Lancet, 384*(9945), 766–781.

2. Marketdata Enterprises Inc. (2012, January 10). Number of American Dieters Soars to 108 Million. [Press Release], Retrieved from http://www.marketdataenterprises.com/wp-content/uploads/2014/01/Diet%20Market%202012%20Forecasts.pdf.

3. 72 developing countries have reached the 2015 MDG 1 target of halving the proportion of hungry people. (2015). Rome: Food and Agriculture Organization of the United Nations. According to the FAO, about 12.9% of the populations of developing countries are undernourished (http://www.fao.org/hunger/key-messages/en/). According to the *Lancet* article above, approximately 32% of the population of developing nations is either overweight or obese.

4. International Diabetes Federation. (2015). *IDF DIABETES ATLAS*, (7th ed., p. 79). Retrieved from http://www.indiaenvironmentportal.org.in/files/file/IDF_Atlas%202015_UK.pdf.

5. Al Humaid, N. (January 2015). Saudi Soft Drinks Market Continues to Fizz. Farrelly & Mitchell Food and Agri-Business Specialists. *Insights.* [Pamphlet]. Retrieved from http://farrellymitchell.com/wp-content/uploads/2015/01/Insights-January-2015-.pdf.

6. Bloom, D. E., Cafiero, E. T., Jané-Llopis, E., Abrahams-Gessel, S., Bloom, L. R., Fathima, . . . Weinstein, C. (2011). The Global Economic Burden of Non-communicable Diseases. Geneva: World Economic Forum, 5. Retrieved from http://www3.weforum.org/docs/WEF_Harvard_HE_GlobalEconomicBurdenNonCommunicableDiseases_2011.pdf.

7. Bloom, D. E., Cafiero, E. T., Jané-Llopis, E., Abrahams-Gessel, S., Bloom, L. R., Fathima, . . . Weinstein, C. (2011).

The Global Economic Burden of Non-communicable Diseases. Geneva: World Economic Forum, 6. Retrieved from http://www3.weforum.org/docs/WEF_Harvard_HE_ GlobalEconomicBurdenNonCommunicableDiseases_2011.pdf.

8. Fildes, A., Charlton, J., Rudisill, C., Littlejohns, P., Prevost, A., & Gulliford, M. (2015). Probability of an obese person attaining normal body weight: Cohort study using electronic health records. *American Journal of Public Health, 105*(9), e54–e59. doi: 10.2105/ AJPH.2015.302773.

9. Marketdata Enterprises Inc. (2011, May 5). Diet Market Worth $60.9 Billion in U.S. Last Year, but Growth Is Flat, Due to the Recession. [Press Release]. Retrieved from http://www.marketdataenterprises. com/wp-content/uploads/2014/01/DietMarket2011PR.pdf.

10. Rand, C. S., & Macgregor, A. M. (1991). Successful weight loss following obesity surgery and the perceived liability of morbid obesity. *International Journal of Obesity, 15*(9), 577.

Chapter 1

1. Casey, B. J., Somerville, L. H., Gotlib, I. H., Ayduk, O., Franklin, N. T., Askren, M. K., . . . Shoda, Y. (2011). (2012). Behavioral and neural correlates of delay of gratification 40 years later. *Proceedings of the National Academy of Sciences of the United States of America, 108* (36),14998–15003. doi:10.1073/pnas.1108561108.

2. Tierney, J. (2011, August 17). Do You Suffer From Decision Fatigue?, *The New York Times Magazine*. Retrieved from http://www.nytimes. com/2011/08/21/magazine/do-you-suffer-from-decision-fatigue. html.

3. Baumeister, R. F., Bratslavsky, E., Muraven, M., & Tice, D. M. (1998). Ego depletion: Is the active self a limited resource? *Journal of Personality and Social Psychology, 74*(5), 1252–1265. doi: 10.1037/0022-3514.74.5.1252.

4. Vohs, K. D., Baumeister, R. F., Schmeichel, B. J., Twenge, J. M., Nelson, N. M., & Tice, D. M. (2008). Making choices impairs subsequent self-control: A limited-resource account of decision making, self-regulation, and active initiative. *Journal of Personality and Social Psychology, 94*(5), 883–898. doi: 10.1037/0022-3514.94.5.883.

5. Danziger, S., Levav, J., Avnaim-Pesso, L., & Kahneman, D. (2011). Extraneous factors in judicial decisions. *Proceedings of the National Academy of Sciences of the United States of America, 108*(17), 6889–6892. doi: 10.1073/pnas.1018033108.

6. Gailliot, M. T., Baumeister, R. F., DeWall, C. N., Maner, J. K., Plant, E. A., Tice, D. M., . . . Schmeichel, B. J. (2007). Self-control relies

on glucose as a limited energy source: Willpower is more than a metaphor. *Journal of Personality and Social Psychology, 92*(2), 325-336. doi: 10.1037/0022-3514.92.2.325.

7. Hofmann, W., Baumeister, R. F., Förster, G., & Vohs, K. D. (2012;2011). Everyday temptations: An experience sampling study of desire, conflict, and self-control. *Journal of Personality and Social Psychology, 102*(6), 1318. doi: 10.1037/a0026545.

8. Baumeister, R. F. (2014). Self-regulation, ego depletion, and inhibition. *Neuropsychologia, 65*, 313–319. doi: 10.1016/j.neuropsychologia.2014.08.0.

9. Gailliot, M. T., & Baumeister, R. F. (2007). The physiology of willpower: Linking blood glucose to self-control. *Personality and Social Psychology Review, 11*(4), 303–327. doi: 10.1177/1088868307303030.

10. McCullough, M. E., & Willoughby, B. L. B. (2009). Religion, self-regulation, and self-control: Associations, explanations, and implications. *Psychological Bulletin, 135*(1), 69–93. doi: 10.1037/a0014213.

11. Luders, E., Toga, A. W., Lepore, N., & Gaser, C. (2009). The underlying anatomical correlates of long-term meditation: Larger hippocampal and frontal volumes of gray matter. *Neuroimage, 45*(3), 672–678. doi: 10.1016/j.neuroimage.2008.12.061.

12. McKellar, J., Stewart, E., & Humphreys, K. (2003). Alcoholics anonymous involvement and positive alcohol-related outcomes: Cause, consequence, or just a correlate? A prospective 2-year study of 2,319 alcohol-dependent men. *Journal of Consulting and Clinical Psychology, 71*(2), 302–308. doi: 10.1037/0022-006X.71.2.302.

13. Greer, S., Goldstein, A., & Walker, M. (2013). The impact of sleep deprivation on food desire in the human brain. *Nature Communications, 4*, 2259. doi: 10.1038/ncomms3259.

14. DeSteno, D., Li, Y., Dickens, L., & Lerner, J. S. (2014). Gratitude: A tool for reducing economic impatience. *Psychological Science, 25*(6), 1262–1267. doi: 10.1177/0956797614529979.

15. Wansink, B., & Sobal, J. (2007). Mindless eating: The 200 daily food decisions we overlook. *Environment and Behavior, 39*(1), 106–123. doi: 10.1177/0013916506295573.

Chapter 2

1. Dulloo, A. G., & Jacquet, J. (1998). Adaptive reduction in basal metabolic rate in response to food deprivation in humans: A role for feedback signals from fat stores. *The American Journal of Clinical Nutrition, 68*(3), 599.

2. Speakman, J. R., & Westerterp, K. R. (2013). A mathematical model of weight loss under total starvation: Evidence against the thrifty-gene hypothesis. *Disease Models & Mechanisms, 6*(1), 236–251. doi: 10.1242/dmm.010009.

3. Rosenkilde, M., Auerbach, P., Reichkendler, M. H., Ploug, T., Stallknecht, B. M., & Sjödin, A. (2012). Body fat loss and compensatory mechanisms in response to different doses of aerobic exercise—a randomized controlled trial in overweight sedentary males. *American Journal of Physiology: Regulatory, Integrative and Comparative Physiology, 303*(6), 571–579. doi: 10.1152/ajpregu.00141.2012.

4. An fMRI shows differences between lean and obese after eating. Puzziferri, N., Zigman, J. M., Thomas, B. P., Mihalakos, P., Gallagher, R., Lutter, M., . . . Tamminga, C. A. (2016). Brain imaging demonstrates a reduced neural impact of eating in obesity. *Obesity, 24*(4), 829-836. doi: 10.1002/oby.21424.

5. Satter, E. M. (2005), *Your Child's Weight: Helping Without Harming,* Madison, WI: Kelsey Press.

6. Wansink, B., Painter, J., & North, J. (2005). Bottomless bowls: Why visual cues of portion size may influence intake. *Obesity Research, 13*(1), 93-100. doi: 10.1038/oby.2005.12.

7. Lisle, D. J., & Goldhamer, A. (2003), *The Pleasure Trap.* Summertown, TN: Healthy Living Publications.

8. Malaisse, W. J., Vanonderbergen, A., Louchami, K., Jijakli, H., & Malaisse-Lagae, F. (1998). Effects of artificial sweeteners on insulin release and cationic fluxes in rat pancreatic islets. *Cellular Signalling, 10*(10), 727–733. doi: 10.1016/S0898-6568(98)00017-5.

9. Malaisse, W. J., Vanonderbergen, A., Louchami, K., Jijakli, H., & Malaisse-Lagae, F. (2011). Intake of high-intensity sweeteners alters the ability of sweet taste to signal caloric consequences: Implications for the learned control of energy and body weight regulation. *The Quarterly Journal of Experimental Psychology, 64*(7), 1430–1441. doi: 10.1080/17470218.2011.552729.

10. Ingalls, A. M., Dickie, M. M., & Snell, G. D. (1996). Obese, a new mutation in the house mouse. *Obesity Research, 4*(1), 101–101. doi: 10.1002/j.1550-8528.1996.tb00519.x.

11. Zhang, Y., Proenca, R., Maffei, M., Barone, M., Leopold, L., & Friedman, J. M. (December 1994). Positional cloning of the mouse obese gene and its human homologue. *Nature, 372*(6505), 425–432. doi: 10.1038/372425a0.

12. Stavro, B. (1995, September 5). With fat-loss drug, Amgen takes on a weighty challenge: Pharmaceuticals: Biotech firm faces much risk and expense in getting the medication from the laboratory to

the marketplace. *Los Angeles Times.* Retrieved from http://articles.
latimes.com/1995-09-05/business/fi-42478_1_fat-drug.

13. Münzberg, H., & Myers, M. G. (2005). Molecular and anatomical
determinants of central leptin resistance. *Nature Neuroscience, 8*(5),
566–570. doi: 10.1038/nn1454.

14. Lustig, R. H. (2006). Childhood obesity: Behavioral aberration
or biochemical drive? Reinterpreting the first law of
thermodynamics. *Nature Clinical Practice Endocrinology &
Metabolism, 2*(8), 447–458. doi: 10.1038/ncpendmet0220.

15. Pinhas-Hamiel, O., Lerner-Geva, L., Copperman, N., & Jacobson, M.
(2007). Lipid and insulin levels in obese children: Changes with age
and puberty. *Obesity, 15,* 2825–2831. doi: 10.1038/oby.2007.335.

16. Grill, H., Schwartz, M., Kaplan, J., Foxhall, J., Breininger, J., & Baskin,
D. (2002). Evidence that the caudal brainstem is a target for the
inhibitory effect of leptin on food intake. *Endocrinology, 143*(1),
239–246. doi: 10.1210/en.143.1.239.

Chapter 3

1. Ng, S., Slining, M., & Popkin, B. (2012). Use of caloric and noncaloric
sweeteners in US consumer packaged foods, 2005–2009. *Journal
of the Academy of Nutrition and Dietetics, 112*(11), 1828–1834. doi:
10.1016/j.jand.2012.07.009.

2. Hanna, J. M., & Hornick, C. A. (1977). Use of coca leaf in southern
Peru: Adaptation or addiction. *Bulletin on Narcotics, 29*(1), 63.

3. Verebey, K., & Gold, M. S. (1988). From coca leaves to crack: The
effects of dose and routes of administration in abuse liability.
Psychiatric Annals, 18, 513–520. doi: 10.3928/0048-5713-19880901-
06.

4. Kenny, P. J., & Johnson, P. M. (2010). Dopamine D2 receptors in
addiction-like reward dysfunction and compulsive eating in obese
rats. *Nature Neuroscience, 13*(5), 635–641. doi: 10.1038/nn.2519.

5. Lenoir, M., Serre, F., Cantin, L., & Ahmed, S. (2007). Intense sweetness
surpasses cocaine reward. *PLOS One, 2*(8), e698. doi:10.1371/journal
.pone.0000698.

6. Hyman, M. (2014). *The Blood Sugar Solution 10-Day Detox Diet.* New
York: Little, Brown and Company, 29.

7. It should be noted that there is variability in the adaptation of rats
to foot shocks. This may require that the subjects be grouped as
sensitive or resistant to foot shocks. For example, see Chen, B. T.,
Yau, H-J, Hatch, C., Kusumoto-Yoshida, I., Cho, S. L., Hopf, F. W.,
& Bonci, A. (2013). Rescuing cocaine-induced prefrontal cortex

hypoactivity prevents compulsive cocaine seeking. *Nature, 496,* 359. doi:10.1038/nature12024.

8. Kenny, P. J., & Johnson, P. M. (2010). Dopamine D2 receptors in addiction-like reward dysfunction and compulsive eating in obese rats. *Nature Neuroscience, 13*(5), 635–641. doi: 10.1038/nn.2519.

9. Kessler, D. A. (2009). *The End of Overeating; Taking Control of the Insatiable American Appetite.* New York: Rodale; Moss, M. (2014). *Salt Sugar Fat: How the Food Giants Hooked Us.* New York: Random House.

10. Bolhuis, D., Costanzo, A., Newman, L., & Keast, R. (2016). Salt promotes passive overconsumption of dietary fat in humans. *Journal of Nutrition, 146*(4), 838-845. doi:10.3945/jn.115.226365.

11. Stice, E., Burger, K., & Yokum, S. (2013). Relative ability of fat and sugar tastes to activate reward, gustatory, and somatosensory regions. *The American Journal of Clinical Nutrition, 98*(6), 1377–1384. doi: 10.3945/ajcn.113.069443.

12. Schulte, E., Avena, N., & Gearhardt, A. (2015). Which foods may be addictive? The roles of processing, fat content, and glycemic load: E0117959. *PLOS One, 10*(2). doi: 10.1371/journal.pone.0117959.

13. Lustig, R. (2012, May 8). The Skinny on Obesity (ep. 4): Sugar—A Sweet Addiction. Retrieved from http://www.uctv.tv/shows/The-Skinny-on-Obesity-Ep-4-Sugar-A-Sweet-Addiction-23717

14. Stewart, J. E., Feinle-Bisset, C., Golding, M., Delahunty, C., Clifton, P. M., & Keast, R. S. J. (2010). Oral sensitivity to fatty acids, food consumption and BMI in human subjects. *British Journal of Nutrition, 104*(1), 145–152. doi: 10.1017/S0007114510000267.

15. Espel, E. (2012, May 8). The Skinny on Obesity (ep. 4): Sugar—A Sweet Addiction. Retrieved from http://www.uctv.tv/shows/The-Skinny-on-Obesity-Ep-4-Sugar-A-Sweet-Addiction-23717; Stice, E., Spoor, S., Bohon, C., Veldhuizen, M. G., & Small, D. M. (2008). Relation of reward from food intake and anticipated food intake to obesity: A functional magnetic resonance imaging study. *Journal of Abnormal Psychology, 117*(4), 924–935. doi: 10.1037/a0013600.

Chapter 4

1. Khokhar, J. Y., Ferguson, C. S., Zhu, A. Z. X., & Tyndale, R. F. (2010). Pharmacogenetics of drug dependence: Role of gene variations in susceptibility and treatment. *Annual Review of Pharmacology and Toxicology, 50*(1), 39–61. doi:10.1146/annurev.pharmtox.010909.105826

2. Hausenblas, H. (2015, November 25). Does the holiday season equal weight gain? *US News & World Report.* Retrieved from http://health .usnews.com/health-news/blogs/eat-run/2015/11/25/does-the-holiday -season-equal-weight-gain.

3. Pursey, K., Stanwell, P., Gearhardt, A., Collins, C., & Burrows, T. (2014). The prevalence of food addiction as assessed by the Yale Food Addiction Scale: A systematic review. *Nutrients, 6*(10), 4552-4590. doi:10.3390/nu6104552.

4. Flagel, S. B., Robinson, T. E., Clark, J. J., Clinton, S. M., Watson, S. J., Seeman, P. ... Akil, H. (2010). An animal model of genetic vulnerability to behavioral disinhibition and responsiveness to reward-related cues: Implications for addiction. *Neuropsychopharmacology, 35*(2), 388–400. doi: 10.1038/npp.2009.142.

5. Flagel, S. B., Watson, S. J., Robinson, T. E., & Akil, H. (2007). Individual differences in the propensity to approach signals vs goals promote different adaptations in the dopamine system of rats. Psychopharmacology, 191(3), 599–607. doi:10.1007/s00213-006-0535-8.

6. Flagel, S. B., Robinson, T. E., Clark, J. J., Clinton, S. M., Watson, S. J., Seeman, P. ... Akil, H. (2010). An animal model of genetic vulnerability to behavioral disinhibition and responsiveness to reward-related cues: Implications for addiction. *Neuropsychopharmacology, 35*(2), 388-400. doi: 10.1038/ npp.2009.142.

7. Lomanowska, A. M., Lovic, V., Rankine, M. J., Mooney, S. J., Robinson, T. E., & Kraemer, G. W. (2011). Inadequate early social experience increases the incentive salience of reward-related cues in adulthood. *Behavioural Brain Research, 220,* 91–99. doi: 10.1016/j.bbr.2011.01.033.

8. Anselme, P., Robinson, M., & Berridge, K. (2013). Reward uncertainty enhances incentive salience attribution as sign-tracking. *Behavioural Brain Research, 238,* 53–61. doi: 10.1016/j.bbr.2012.10.006.

Chapter 5

1. Gazzaniga, M. S. (1967). The split brain in man. *Scientific American, 217*(2), 24–29. doi: 10.1038/scientificamerican0867-24.

2. Gazzaniga, M. S. (2011). *Who's in charge?: Free will and the science of the brain* (1st ed.). New York: HarperCollins, 82.

3. Gazzaniga, M. S., & LeDoux, J. E. (1978). *The integrated mind.* New York: Plenum Press.

4. Bem, D. J. (1972). Self-perception theory. *Advances in Experimental Social Psychology, 6,* 2–62.

Chapter 6

1. Li, Y., Burrows, N., Gregg, E., Albright, A., & Geiss, L. (2012). Declining rates of hospitalization for nontraumatic lower-extremity amputation in the diabetic population aged 40 years or older: U.S., 1988–2008. *Diabetes Care, 35*(2), 273–277. doi: 10.2337/dc11-1360; http://www.diabetes.org/diabetes-basics/statistics/.

2. Baumeister, R. F. & Toerney, J. (2011). *Willpower: Rediscovering the greatest human strength.* New York: Penguin Group.

3. While artificial sweeteners stimulate the taste buds, they also affect the brain. Aspartame, for example can reduce the production of dopamine. Humphries, P., Pretorius, E. & Naudé, H. (2008). They are both direct and indirect cellular effects of aspartame on the brain. *European Journal of Clinical Nutrition, 62*(4), 451–462. doi: 10.1038/sj.ejcn.1602866). The lack of a nutrient reward when saccharin is tasted results in reduced dopamine surges after conditioning. Mark, G. P., Blander, D. S., & Hoebel, B. G. (1991). A conditioned stimulus decreases extracellular dopamine in the nucleus accumbens after the development of a learned taste aversion. *Brain Research, 551*(1), 308–310. doi: 10.1016/0006-8993(91)90946-S). Like the artificial sweeteners, stevia is nonnutritive and may cause long-term depressed levels of dopamine.

4. Suez, J., Korem, T., Zeevi, D., Zilberman-Schapira, G., Thaiss, C., Maza, O., . . . Elinav, (2014). Artificial sweeteners induce glucose intolerance by altering the gut microbiota. *Nature, 514*(7521), 181. doi:10.1038/nature13793.

5. Wang, Q-P. et al. (2016) Sucralose promotes food intake through NPY and a neuronal fasting response. *Cell Metabolism, 24*(1), 75–90.

6. Juntunen, K., Niskanen, L., Liukkonen, K., Poittanen, K., Holst, J., & Mykkanen, H. (2002). Postprandial glucose, insulin, and incretin responses to grain products in healthy subjects. *The American Journal of Clinical Nutrition, 75*(2), 254.

7. Schulte, E., Avena, N., & Gearhardt, A. (2015). Which foods may be addictive? The roles of processing, fat content, and glycemic load: E0117959. *PLOS One, 10*(2) doi: 10.1371/journal.pone.0117959.

8. Reid, K., Baron, K., & Zee, P. (2014). Meal timing influences daily caloric intake in healthy adults. *Nutrition Research, 34*(11), 930-935. doi:10.1016/j.nutres.2014.09.010.

9. Gill, S., & Panda, S. (2015). A smartphone app reveals erratic diurnal eating patterns in humans that can be modulated for health benefits. *Cell Metabolism, 22*(5), 789-798. doi:10.1016/j.cmet.2015.09.005.

10. Alirezaei, M., Kemball, C. C., Flynn, C. T., Wood, M. R., Whitton, J. L., & Kiosses, W. B. (2010). Short-term fasting induces profound neuronal autophagy. *Autophagy, 6*(6), 702–710. doi: 10.4161/auto.6.6.12376

11. Marinac, C. R., Nelson, S. H., Breen, C. I., Hartman, S. J., Natarajan, L., Pierce, J. P., . . . Patterson, R. E. (2016). Prolonged nightly fasting and breast cancer prognosis. *JAMA Oncology, 2*(8), 1049.

12. Parks, E., & McCrory, M. (2005). When to eat and how often? *American Journal of Clinical Nutrition, 81*(1), 3-4.

13. Kahleova, H., Belinova, L., Malinska, H., Oliyarnyk, O., Trnovska, J., Skop, V., . . . Pelikanova, T. (2014). Eating two larger meals a day (breakfast and lunch) is more effective than six smaller meals in a reduced-energy regimen for patients with type 2 diabetes: A randomised crossover study. *Diabetologia, 57*(8), 1552–1560. doi: 10.1007/s00125-014-3253-5.

Chapter 7

1. Lally, P., Van Jaarsveld, C., Potts, H., & Wardle, J. (2010). How are habits formed: Modelling habit formation in the real world. *European Journal of Social Psychology, 40*(6), 998–1009. doi: 10.1002/ejsp.674.

2. Pilcher, J., Morris, D., Donnelly, J., & Feigl, H. (2015). Interactions between sleep habits and self-control. *Frontiers in Human Neuroscience, 9,* 284. doi: 10.3389/fnhum.2015.00284.

3. Erickson, K. I., Voss, M. W., Prakash, R. S., Basak, C., Szabo, A., Chaddock, L., . . . Gage, F. (2011). Exercise training increases size of hippocampus and improves memory. *Proceedings of the National Academy of Sciences of the United States of America, 108*(7), 3017–3022. http://doi.org/10.1073/pnas.1015950108.

4. Erickson, K., Weinstein, A., & Lopez, O. (2012). Physical activity, brain plasticity, and Alzheimer's disease. *Archives of Medical Research, 43*(8), 615–621. doi: 10.1016/j.arcmed.2012.09.008.

5. Walsh, N., Gleeson, M., Pyne, D., Nieman, D., Dhabhar, F., Shephard, R., . . . Kajeniene, A. (2011). Position statement. Part two: Maintaining immune health. *Exercise Immunology Review, 17,* 64.

6. Kemmler, W., Lauber, D., Weineck, J., Hensen, J., Kalender, W., & Engelke, K. (2004). Benefits of 2 years of intense exercise on bone density, physical fitness, and blood lipids in early postmenopausal osteopenic women. *Archives of Internal Medicine, 164*(10), 1084.

7. Elavsky, S. (2010). Longitudinal examination of the exercise and self-esteem model in middle-aged women. *Journal of Sport & Exercise Psychology, 32*(6), 862–880.

8. Penhollow, T. M. & Young, M. (2004). Sexual desirability and sexual performance: Does exercise and fitness really matter? *Electronic Journal of Human Sexuality, 7.* http://www.ejhs.org/volume7/fitness.html.

9. Mikus, C. R., Blair, S. N., Earnest, C. P., Martin, C. K., Thompson, A. M., & Church, T. S. (2009). Changes in weight, waist circumference and compensatory responses with different doses of exercise among sedentary, overweight postmenopausal women. *PlOS One, 4*(2), e4515. doi: 10.1371/journal.pone.0004515.

10. Fothergill, E., Guo, J., Howard, L., Kerns, J. C., Knuth, N. D., Brychta, R., . . . Hall, K. D. (2016). Persistent metabolic adaptation 6 years after "The biggest loser" competition. *Obesity, 24*(8), 1612-1619. doi: 10.1002/oby.21538.

11. Larson-Meyer, D., Redman, L., Heilbronn, L., Martin, C., & Ravussin, E. (2010). Caloric restriction with or without exercise: The fitness versus fatness debate. *Medicine and Science in Sports and Exercise, 42*(1), 152.

Chapter 8

1. Greene, A. (2011, July 18). 7 things you didn't know about your taste buds. *Woman's Day.* Retrieved from http://www.womansday.com/health-fitness/wellness/a5789/7-things-you-didnt-know-about-your-taste-buds-119709/.

2. Badman, M. K., & Flier, J. S. (2005). The gut and energy balance: Visceral allies in the obesity wars. *Science, 307*(5717), 1909–1914. doi: 10.1126/science.110995.

3. Following the BLE weight-loss plan typically results in weight-loss rates of one to three pounds per week. This rate is considered desirable. Blackburn, G. (1995). Effect of degree of weight loss on health benefits. *Obesity Research, 3,* 211S-216S. Regarding the 10% figure, see: National Institutes of Health (U.S.), NHLBI Obesity Education Initiative, North American Association for the Study of Obesity, & National Heart, Lung, and Blood Institute. (2000). *The practical guide: Identification, evaluation, and treatment of overweight and obesity in adults.* Bethesda, MD.: National Institutes of Health, National Heart, Lung, and Blood Institute, NHLBI Obesity Education Initiative, North American Association for the Study of Obesity.

4. Voelker, R. (2015). Partially hydrogenated oils are out. *JAMA, 314*(5), 443.

5. An example of the lack of consensus may be found in the study: Schwingshackl, L., & Hoffmann, G. (2013). Comparison of effects of long-term low-fat vs high-fat diets on blood lipid levels in overweight or obese patients: A systematic review and meta-

analysis. *Journal of the Academy of Nutrition and Dietetics, 113*(12), 1640–1661. doi: 10.1016/j.jand.2013.07.010.

6. Reynolds, R. M., Padfield, P. L., & Seckl, J. R. (2006). Disorders of sodium balance. *BMJ: British Medical Journal, 332*(7543), 702–705. doi: 10.1136/bmj.332.7543.702.

7. Campbell, T. C., Campbell, T. M., (2006). *The China study: The most comprehensive study of nutrition ever conducted and the startling implications for diet, weight loss, and long-term health.* (1st BenBella Books ed.) Dallas, TX: BenBella Books.

8. World Cancer Research Fund/American Institute for Cancer Research. (2007). *Food, nutrition, physical activity, and the prevention of cancer: A global perspective.* Washington, DC: AICR, 117.

Chapter 9

1. Hwang, K. O., Ottenbacher, A. J., Green, A. P., Cannon-Diehl, M. R., Richardson, O., Bernstam, E. V., & Thomas, E. J. (2010). Social support in an internet weight loss community. *International Journal of Medical Informatics, 79*(1), 5–13. doi: 10.1016/j. ijmedinf.2009.10.003.

2. The National Weight Control Registry, accessed on March 28, 2016. http://www.nwcr.ws/.

3. Kreitzman, S. N., Coxon, A. Y., & Szaz, K. F. (1992). Glycogen storage: Illusions of easy weight loss, excessive weight regain, and distortions in estimates of body composition. *The American Journal of Clinical Nutrition, 56*(1 Suppl.), 292S.

4. Pacanowski, C. R., & Levitsky, D. A. (2015). Frequent self-weighing and visual feedback for weight loss in overweight adults. *Journal of Obesity, 2015*, 1–9. doi: 10.1155/2015/763680.

Chapter 10

1. For references of the power of prayer and meditation to replenish willpower, see: McCullough, M. E., & Willoughby, B. L. B. (2009). Religion, self-regulation, and self-control: Associations, explanations, and implications. *Psychological Bulletin, 135*(1), 69–93. doi: 10.1037/a0014213; and Baumeister, R. F., & Tierney, J. (2011). *Willpower: Rediscovering the greatest human strength.* New York: Penguin Group, 180.

2. Luders, E., Cherbuin, N., & Kurth, F. (2015). Forever young(er): Potential age-defying effects of long-term meditation on gray matter atrophy. *Frontiers in Psychology, 5:1551.* doi: 10.3389/fpsyg.2014.01551.

3. Brewer, J. A., Worhunsky, P. D., Gray, J. R., Tang, Y., Weber, J., & Kober, H. (2011). Meditation experience is associated with differences in default mode network activity and connectivity. *Proceedings of the National Academy of Sciences of the United States of America, 108*(50), 20254–20259. http://doi.org/10.1073/pnas.1112029108.

4. Goyal, M., Singh, S., Sibinga, E. M. S., Gould, N. F., Rowland-Seymour, A., Sharma, R., . . . Haythornthwaite, J. A. (2014). Meditation programs for psychological stress and well-being: A systematic review and meta-analysis. *JAMA Internal Medicine, 174*(3), 357–368. doi: 10.1001/jamainternmed.2013.13018.

5. Mrazek, M. D., Franklin, M. S., Phillips, D. T., Baird, B., & Schooler, J. W. (2013). Mindfulness training improves working memory capacity and GRE performance while reducing mind wandering. *Psychological Science, 24*(5), 776–781.

6. Tang, Y., Tang, R., & Posner, M. I. (2013). Brief meditation training induces smoking reduction. *Proceedings of the National Academy of Sciences of the United States of America, 110*(34), 13971–13975. doi: 10.1073/pnas.1311887110.

7. Barnes, V. A., Davis, H. C., Murzynowski, J. B., & Treiber, F. A. (2004). Impact of meditation on resting and ambulatory blood pressure and heart rate in youth. *Psychosomatic Medicine, 66*(6), 909–914. doi: 10.1097/01.psy.0000145902.91749.35.

8. Schienker, B. R., Dlugolecki, D. W., & Doherty, K. (1994). The impact of self-presentations on self-appraisals and behavior: The power of public commitment. *Personality and Social Psychology Bulletin, 20*(1), 20–33. doi: 10.1177/0146167294201002.

9. Nyer, P. U., & Dellande, S. (2010). Public commitment as a motivator for weight loss. *Psychology and Marketing, 27*(1), 1–12. doi: 10.1002/mar.20316.

10. Seligman, M. (2011). Find three good things each day. Retrieved from http://www.actionforhappiness.org/take-action/find-three-good-things-each-day

11. Kazdin, A. E. (1974). Reactive self-monitoring: The effects of response desirability, goal setting, and feedback. *Journal of Consulting and Clinical Psychology, 42*(5), 704–716. doi: 10.1037/h0037050.

12. Baumeister, R. F., DeWall, C. N., Ciarocco, N. J., & Twenge, J. M. (2005). Social exclusion impairs self-regulation. *Journal of Personality and Social Psychology, 88*(4), 589–604. doi: 10.1037/0022-3514.88.4.589.

13. McCullough, M. E., & Willoughby, B. L. B. (2009). Religion, self-regulation, and self-control: Associations, explanations, and implications. *Psychological Bulletin, 135*(1), 69–93. doi: 10.1037/a0014213.

14. McGonigal, K. (2012). *The willpower instinct: How self-control works, why it matters, and what you can do to get more of it.* New York: Penguin Group, 25.

15. DeSteno, D., Li, Y., Dickens, L., & Lerner, J. S. (2014). Gratitude: A tool for reducing economic impatience. *Psychological Science, 25*(6), 1262–1267. doi: 10.1177/0956797614529979.

16. Gray, K. (2010). Moral transformation: Good and evil turn the weak into the mighty. *Social Psychological and Personality Science, 1*(3), 253–258. doi: 10.1177/1948550610367686.

17. Hill, N. (1937). *Think and grow rich.* Meriden, CT: The Ralston Society.

Chapter 11

1. National Research Council (U.S.). Committee on National Monitoring of Human Tissues. (1991). *Monitoring human tissues for toxic substances.* Washington, DC: National Academy Press, 64.

2. Lim, J., Son, H., Park, S., Jacobs, D., & Lee, D. (2011). Inverse associations between long-term weight change and serum concentrations of persistent organic pollutants. *International Journal of Obesity, 35*(5), 744–747. doi: 10.1038/ijo.2010.188.

3. Dulloo, A. G., & Jacquet, J. (1998). Adaptive reduction in basal metabolic rate in response to food deprivation in humans: A role for feedback signals from fat stores. *The American Journal of Clinical Nutrition, 68*(3), 599.

4. Sumithran, P., Prendergast, L. A., Delbridge, E., Purcell, K., Shulkes, A., Kriketos, A., & Proietto, J. (2011). Long-term persistence of hormonal adaptations to weight loss. *The New England Journal of Medicine, 365*(17), 1597–1604. doi: 10.1056/NEJMoa1105816.

5. Satter, E. (2007). Eating competence: Definition and evidence for the Satter eating competence model. *Journal of Nutrition Education and Behavior, 39*(5), S142–S153. doi: 10.1016/j.jneb.2007.01.006.

6. Kenny, P. J., & Johnson, P. M. (2010). Dopamine D2 receptors in addiction-like reward dysfunction and compulsive eating in obese rats. *Nature Neuroscience, 13*(5), 635–641. doi: 10.1038/nn.2519.

7. Satter, E., (2008). *Secrets of feeding a healthy family: How to eat, how to raise good eaters, how to cook.* Madison, WI: Kelcy Press, 82.

8. Camilleri, M., Colemont, L., Phillips, S., Brown, M., Thomforde, G., Chapman, N., & Zinsmeister, A. (1989). Human gastric emptying and colonic filling of solids characterized by a new method. *The American Journal of Physiology, 257*(2, Pt. 1), G284.

Chapter 12

1. Wing, R. R., & Phelan, S. (2005). Long-term weight loss maintenance. *The American Journal of Clinical Nutrition, 82*(1 Suppl.), 222S.

Chapter 13

1. Herman, C. P., & Mack, D. (1975). Restrained and unrestrained eating. *Journal of Personality, 43*(4), 647.

Chapter 14

1. There are many "ideal weight" formulas, and you can find them online. One of the earliest was provided by Broca P. P., (1871/1877). *Mémoires d'anthropologie.* Paris, the same Dr. Broca who discovered Broca's area. It is approximately 100 pounds (women) or 110 pounds (men) for the first 60 inches (5 feet) of height plus 5 pounds for each inch above that. To cover variations in body composition, Broca suggested that the desirable weight would be within 15 percent of the calculated number.

2. Satter, E. (2007). Eating competence: Definition and evidence for the Satter eating competence model. *Journal of Nutrition Education and Behavior, 39*(5), S142–S153. doi: 10.1016/j.jneb.2007.01.006.

Chapter 15: Conclusion

1. Popa, T. & Ladea, M. (2012). Nutrition and depression at the forefront of progress. *Journal of Medicine and Life, 5*(4), 414–419.

2. White, B., Horwath, C., & Conner, T. (2013). Many apples a day keep the blues away—daily experiences of negative and positive affect and food consumption in young adults. *British Journal of Health Psychology, 18*(4), 782.

3. Gomez-Pinilla, F., & Nguyen, T. T. J. (2012). Natural mood foods: The actions of polyphenols against psychiatric and cognitive disorders. *Nutritional Neuroscience, 15*(3), 127.

4. Mujcic, R., & Oswald, A. J. (2016), Evolution of well-being and happiness after increases in consumption of fruit and vegetables. *American Journal of Public Health, 106*(8), 1504–1510.

5. Chang, C., Ke, D., & Chen, J. (2009). Essential fatty acids and human brain. *Acta Neurologica Taiwanica, 18*(4), 231.

6. Simopoulos, A. P. (2002). The importance of the ratio of omega-6/omega-3 essential fatty acids. *Biomedicine & Pharmacotherapy, 56*(8), 365–379. doi: 10.1016/S0753-3322(02)00253-6.

7. Russo, G. L. (2009). Dietary n-6 and n-3 polyunsaturated fatty acids: From biochemistry to clinical implications in cardiovascular prevention. *Biochemical Pharmacology, 77*(6), 937–946. doi: 10.1016/j .bcp.2008.10.020.

8. Stangl, D., & Thuret, S. (2009). Impact of diet on adult hippocampal neurogenesis. *Genes and Nutrition, 4*(4), 271–282. doi: 10.1007/ s12263-009-0134-5.

9. Baumeister, R., & Tierney, J. (2011). *Willpower: Rediscovering the greatest human strength*. New York: Penguin Press, 136.

10. Lowe, M. R., Kral, T. V. E., & Miller-Kovach, K. (2008). Weight-loss maintenance 1, 2 and 5 years after successful completion of a weight-loss programme. *British Journal of Nutrition, 99*(4), 925–930. doi: 10.1017/S0007114507862416; Chaudhry, Z. W., Clark, J. M., Doshi, R. S., Gudzune, K. A., Jacobs, D. K., Mehta, A. K., et al. (2015). Efficacy of commercial weight-loss programs: An updated systematic review. *Annals of Internal Medicine, 162*(7), 501. doi: 10.7326/M14-2238.

11. Rock, C. L., Flatt, S. W., Sherwood, N. E., Karanja, N., Pakiz, B., & Thomson, C. A. (2010). Effect of a free prepared meal and incentivized weight loss program on weight loss and weight loss maintenance in obese and overweight women: A randomized controlled trial. *JAMA, 304*(16), 1803–1810. doi: 10.1001/jama.2010.1503.

INDEX

ACKNOWLEDGMENTS

I expect my editor will tell me my acknowledgments are too long, but I don't care. If the book can be hundreds of pages, surely more than one or two can be spared to express the depth of gratitude I feel for all who have contributed, in ways both momentous and momentary, to this extraordinary thing called Bright Line Eating. It is, after all, more than a book; it is a movement.

So I must thank . . .

First, the Bright Line Eaters themselves, the founders, the ones who signed up at the beginning. Thank you for taking the plunge. I'm so grateful for your trust in me and so impressed by the willingness, fervor, and devotion with which you've learned this way of life, applied it, and used it to break free. You are the reason my feet hit the floor in the morning.

My precious Bright Lifers, who have chosen to stay close to the Mothership after the Boot Camp ends. It takes my breath away how much love and support you pour into our community and into my heart. When I struggle, I bring it to you and you carry me. Thank you for letting me be human. I am humbled that I get to be a Bright Lifer with you and beyond privileged to coach you in the ongoing, magical dance of maintenance.

The tribe! The hundreds of thousands of people who have taken the Susceptibility Quiz, read the free report, signed up for updates from the Bright Line Eating e-mail list, tried the 14-Day Challenge, enrolled in the Boot Camp, journeyed through Bright Line Healing and Bright Line Mind, attended the annual Bright Line Eating Family Reunion, watched the weekly VLOGs, left comments, sent in feedback, and spread the word. Thank you for being on board, for being brilliant, and for showing me so much love.

My Magnificent Mavens Mastermind Group: Linden Morris Delrio, Marianne Marsh, and Cathy Cox. Thank you so much for the depth and constancy of your support and unconditional love. We have created something truly extraordinary out of our 90-minute haven each week. I could not do what I do on any level without you.

My incredible team here at Bright Line Eating. Incredible. Mind-blowingly, shout-it-from-the-rooftops *incredible*. Online entrepreneurs are always griping about their issues with their team. Not me. Having a team is the *best* part, not the hardest part. The dedication, ownership, passion, loyalty, creativity, consistency, and brilliance you all bring to our mission blows me away every single day. When I started this, I never imagined having one employee, let alone dozens, but you have become, in many ways, the focal point of my life. There are no words to express how much you mean to me. I am committed to striving to make Bright Line Eating *the best place to work on earth* until I drop. For you. Steven Gomez, Chris Davis, Julia Harold, Jenn Moon, Linden Morris Delrio, Marianne Marsh, Tracy Stroh, David Lewis, Simone Simms, Arianna Hillis, Lynn Coulston, Crystal Gomez, Kaitlyn Moon, Bill Wilson, Nadia Briones, Jeff Pehrson, Lori Lang, Tara Bogdon, Erica Stuart, Angela Simpson, Gretchen Stoll, and Laura Carr, I bow before you in gratitude. Can you believe what we've created together? And how much *fun* it's been? I friggin' love you so much I can't stand it! And to all the future BLE team members, know that I welcome you, I love you, and I'm so grateful you've chosen to add your brilliance to the mix. The best is yet to come.

The research team who made this book possible: Nancy Wolf, Ph.D.; Nathan Denkin, Ph.D.; Jonathan Iuzzini; and Ruth Washam. Thank you for your prodigious efforts to crunch the numbers in time. And Jeanne Hurlbert and Win Guon of Hurlbert Consulting Group for revamping our research program and busily amassing data that shows that Bright Line Eating is the most successful weight loss program on earth by far. You do the most important and the least acknowledged work at Bright Line Eating and I'm so very grateful for your brilliance and expertise. Our future will be built on your shoulders.

Andrew Kurt Thaw, Ph.D., and Sabrina Grondhuis, Ph.D., for writing and submitting the very first scientific paper on the Bright Line Eating program. Thank you for believing in what we're doing here at BLE and helping us get the word out.

Our phenomenal House Leaders and VIP Posters, you make our Online Support Community extraordinary—a haven for profound healing and transformation. You channel and embody the love we stand for here at Bright Line Eating and bring the care and acceptance that are so critical to our Boot Campers' success. Michelle Elsbree, a hug and a sweet thank you for your important service, and Johannes Bockwoldt of Take On Film Productions, thank you for bringing the Food Freedom videos to life.

The luminaries who mentored this academic and helped her build a platform for her ideas. Jeff Walker, I am so very lucky that Product Launch Formula appeared right when I was searching online for a road map, and that I somehow knew to just keep my head down and *follow it.* Thank you for staying true to your calling and, by extension, impacting all the people who now get to hear about Bright Line Eating who wouldn't have otherwise. I am grateful for the blessing of being in your Platinum Plus Mastermind Group with some of the most huge-hearted, brilliant, fun, generous people out there, and I pinch myself every day that this is the company I keep.

Ryan Eliason, yours was the first online course I ever took, and it laid the foundation strong and true. You taught me how to have a business plan and a success plan, and that being in business doesn't have to be incongruous with changing the world. I'll never forget the day you told me that I wasn't building a business, I was starting a movement. It was a lightbulb moment.

Sage Lavine, I feel so lucky to be soul sisters with you on this improbable, fantastical journey of feminine entrepreneurship. Thank you for teaching me what it takes to be a leader. Your example of self-care, conscious life-crafting, and dedicated service illumines a path for me and so many others to follow. Spring cleaning with you is the antidote to every difficulty.

Justin Livingston, the playful genius, I will forever strive to be in the room when you speak. You had my back right from the beginning. Thank you for thinking as deeply as you do about the things that really matter.

Annie Pratt, you are a leadership mentor extraordinaire. Your wisdom informs what we do here at Bright Line Eating Solutions, LLC on every level. You taught me how to organize my business, how to create a psychologically safe environment where everyone feels like they can surface challenging issues, and how to let my leaders shine. Our entire team is so enriched by your experienced guidance. Thank you for being glorious you.

My coaches Clive Prout and Monica Leggett. Clive, you have watched my food journey nearly from the beginning, and your steady, gentle questioning cuts to the heart of every matter. Thank you for calling me to a higher standard of life crafting. You are the person by whom I most enjoy being heard. Monica, I would not have weathered this crazy storm without you. We've been through the whole improbable arc together, and somehow one conversation with you can take the most intractable jumble of commitments and lay them out straight and smooth and ready to be conquered.

My affiliate partners. You are so badass, so brilliant, and up to such amazing stuff in this world. I get to share your awesomeness with my tribe, and you share about Bright Line Eating with yours, and together we make the world a better place. You believed in me right from the beginning. Thank you for that. We would not have been able to get the word out without each and every one of you.

And then the Robbins family. I mean, where do I begin? Ocean Robbins, you astound me with your integrity, wisdom, insight, and fair-mindedness. I trust you as much as I trust anyone on this earth; it's unbelievable what an amazing person you are, what a visionary leader, and what a good friend. Thank you for plucking me out of obscurity and offering your incomparable partnership and mentorship on this journey. And John, the budding connection we have is a bright light in my life. Thank you for writing a beautiful foreword for this book, and placing the Bright Line Eating movement in the historical context of the entire Food Revolution, for which you have been, and continue to be, such a pivotal leader.

I love you and Deo and Phoenix, and feel grateful to have been welcomed into your family so lovingly.

Lucinda Blumenfeld, my agent extraordinaire, you are not only a phenomenal, super-skilled agent, but also a friend and lady. You always make me smile. I'm so grateful to have you in my corner and, as a first-time author, I have to say it's just such a treat to adore your agent so much. I pinch myself.

Patty Gift. Thank you for watching my Food Freedom videos and loving them. Thank you for believing in me and in this project. Learning that you wanted, not only for Hay House to publish my book but to *edit it yourself* was one of the peak moments of my life. And you are such a delight to work with; how could I not adore you?

Reid Tracy, Sally Mason-Swaab, and all the folks at Hay House, I have so much respect for the culture of your company and what you're up to in the world, publishing books that really matter, books that change people's lives. Reid, thank you for always having my back—for real—and for being a gentleman and wise mentor. The other publishing companies fail to follow your lead in the online marketing space at their peril. You have got it going on over at Hay House.

Cinzia Damonte, you drew the most haunting, beautiful illustrations for this book. The first time I saw your art my jaw dropped and my heart melted. This book sits differently in one's hands because of the quality and care of your drawings. Thank you.

The fourteen people who volunteered to proofread the book, or portions of the book, at critical junctures: Karen Van Meenen, Janine de Villiers, Julia Galbus, Ginny Freyer, Joseph Fleischman (my dad!), Eileen Lass, Sharon Cheek, Sunny St. Pierre, Jackie Montara, Dr. Andrew Kurt Thaw, Chris Davis, Chris Foti, Benjamin Schaefer, and Jenn Moon. You caught so many typos it makes me shudder. Thank you for your generous service and sharp eyes.

And now the two people without whom this book absolutely, positively could not, would not, exist, at least not in this decade: Dr. Nathan Denkin and Nicola Kraus. Nat, you chased down hundreds upon hundreds of references for studies I'd heard described at some conference years ago, or statistics I'd bandied about at dinner parties, whose source I couldn't rightly recall. Thank you for your prodigious efforts, and for your protective spirit. You chose to dedicate a huge chunk of your life to making sure that every word is true, factual, and substantiated. I cannot express my gratitude. And lovely Marilyn, thank you for loaning him to me for this project. Your sacrifice has not gone unnoticed.

Nicola Kraus, your partnership in the creation of this work has been unparalleled. I'm so glad I was tipped off (thanks, Lucinda!) that, with my schedule, I should bring you on as my writing coach, and so much more. What we have created here, thanks to you, is exactly, precisely, what I'd hoped it would be. I will remember, to my dying day, cozying up in your Brooklyn office, side by side, to map out the sections and paragraphs of this book. Thank you for the breakfast apples and toasted pecans, for the disco-ball ceiling light in your guest bedroom, and for your endless hospitality, grace, service, wit, optimism, wise counsel, and thoughtful gifts. You are a dream. And David and Sophie, thanks for lending mom to this project. It wouldn't have happened without her.

Ashley Bernardi, because of Ron Friedman I already knew you were a PR rock star goddess, but what I didn't expect was what an amazing friend you would turn out to be, and how you would hold my hand for every TV appearance. I adore you! Sharon Bially from Book Savvy PR, you are an incredible addition to our PR team, and I feel so excited and blessed that I found you and that you and Ashley work so well together. Thank you both for getting the word out to everyone who needs this information. None of this hard work matters if no one hears about it.

Mat Miller, I cannot express how grateful I am that you rescued us from near-fatal demise. Your integrity and wise counsel truly saved the day. Anyone hoping their book launch will be a success needs to retain your services, pronto. And Krista, if every business owner had support like yours, the world would finally function well.

To all the friends and mentors in 12-Step recovery, thank you for saving my life . . . and then showing me what to do with it. Your grace and wisdom lay the foundation for these pages. I couldn't live without you, literally, and my heart bursts with the reality that I wouldn't want to. Everything I have, do, or am, is because of you, and I live my life in service of our collective purpose.

And, of course, ultimately, I could not have done any of this without the love and support of my extraordinary friends and family. I guess everyone thinks this, but I truly have the best besties in the world, folks who make this crazy journey called life something worth waking up to every day. Shiraz Nerenberg, Shira Coleman, Cathy Cox, Diane O'Heron, Lionel Church, Ari Whitten, Jon Iuzzini, Ron Friedman, Beth Wilson, Pat Kress, Gabe Enz, Robin Kulibert, Emily Brightman, Dana Oliver, Jenn Moon, Molly Larkin, Benjamin Schaefer, Darcy Shepherd, Marianne Marsh, Linden Morris Delrio, Chris Davis, Tracy Stroh, Julia Harold, Steven Gomez, Jeff Pehrson, Arin Wiscomb, Ian Ferguson, Katie Mae, Amy Fortoul, Pat Reynolds, Georgia Whitney, Khieta Davis, Amy Grigg, Erica Stuart, Marie Coppola, Bob & Debbie Rosenfeld, Glenn Egli, Jose DaCosta, and Mary Kay Osborne, you lift me up, hold me up, and patch me up. Thank you for being willing to hear the long version of every story.

My parents, Mariah Perkins and Joseph Fleischman. My mom. My dad. I'm able to show up for this whole thing because of you. Throughout my childhood you were there with devoted, open, honest, unconditional love and because of that I became someone who could throw herself into the arms of the universe, trusting it would catch her. Thank you for teaching me to be honest, always, and giving me space to share what's real. I love you. You are my biggest cheerleaders and the first two people I want to call when life gets interesting. And to my in-laws, Hubert and Liliane Thompson, and my stepparents, Gary Wolk and Emily Porzia, thank you for your love and support all along the way.

Which brings me to my husband, David, and our girls. David, you know this book wouldn't exist without you. The sweetness and constancy of your love for me take my breath away. I truly believe that you are a gift straight from God to me. I don't know anybody steadier, wiser, or more incisive at critical moments. Nor wittier. Holy smokes you're funny! Thank goodness you're at the helm, steadying the Bright Line Eating ship—we are such a great team. Thank you for stepping into the magical new world of our post-Labor Day love. It is a privilege to be partnered with you, in this world, and all the worlds to come.

And my sweet, precious daughters: Zoe, Alexis, and Maya. As you age and you realize how much time Mommy took to do this and how much of that came from your childhood, I just hope it feels worth it to you. I hope that, by example, you will come to know that whatever you dream of, you can create it, build it, and achieve it; that any Big Hairy Audacious Goal that lands in your heart is worth pursuing and pursuing all out. I am so proud of the girls you are and the young women you're becoming, and I love you with every breath I take.

And above all, God. My gratitude knows no bounds. You perform everything that is appointed for me, and perfect everything that concerns me. I make no claim to understanding your unknowable essence, but I rest in your sweet shelter, always, and your praise is the whisper behind every word.

What a world it would be if every human being could experience the miracle of watching their deepest pain, their most prolonged suffering, their most tragic and ridiculous struggle turned into a service they can perform that helps other people. My personal belief is that Bright Line Eating continues to spread as rapidly as it does because millions of people are praying for a solution every single day, beseeching God for help, and it's those prayers that are fashioning this movement, fueling the creation of this whole enterprise, and it's in service of those desperate yearnings that I get to keep waking up in the morning. I just pray to be worthy of the task.

ABOUT THE AUTHOR

Susan Peirce Thompson, Ph.D., is an Adjunct Associate Professor of Brain and Cognitive Sciences at the University of Rochester and an expert in the psychology of eating. She is President of the Institute for Sustainable Weight Loss and the founder and CEO of Bright Line Eating Solutions, a company dedicated to helping people achieve long-term, sustainable weight loss. Her program utilizes cutting-edge research to explain how the brain blocks weight loss and every day she teaches people how to undo that damage so they can live Happy, Thin, and Free. She lives in Pittsford, New York, with her husband and their three daughters.

We hope you enjoyed this Hay House book. If you'd like to receive our online catalog featuring additional information on Hay House books and products, or if you'd like to find out more about the Hay Foundation, please contact:

Hay House, Inc., P.O. Box 5100, Carlsbad, CA 92018-5100
(760) 431-7695 or (800) 654-5126
(760) 431-6948 (fax) or (800) 650-5115 (fax)
www.hayhouse.com® • www.hayfoundation.org

———

Published in Australia by:
Hay House Australia Pty. Ltd., 18/36 Ralph St., Alexandria NSW 2015
Phone: 612-9669-4299 • *Fax:* 612-9669-4144 • www.hayhouse.com.au

Published in the United Kingdom by:
Hay House UK, Ltd., Astley House, 33 Notting Hill Gate, London W11 3JQ
Phone: 44-20-3675-2450 • *Fax:* 44-20-3675-2451 • www.hayhouse.co.uk

Published in India by: Hay House Publishers India,
Muskaan Complex, Plot No. 3, B-2, Vasant Kunj, New Delhi 110 070
Phone: 91-11-4176-1620 • *Fax:* 91-11-4176-1630 • www.hayhouse.co.in

———

Access New Knowledge.
Anytime. Anywhere.

Learn and evolve at your own pace
with the world's leading experts.

www.hayhouseU.com